EXPECTING IN THE ER

TINA BECKETT

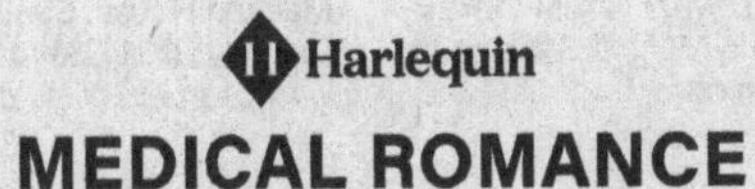

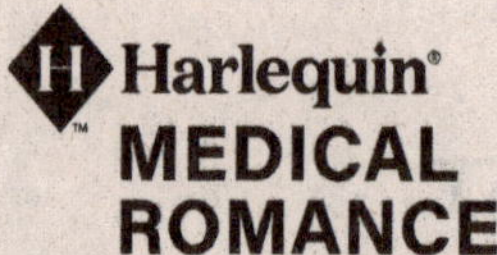

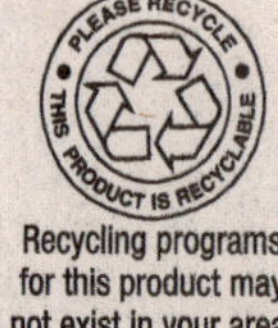

Recycling programs for this product may not exist in your area

ISBN-13: 978-1-335-99365-6

Expecting in the ER

For questions and comments about the quality of this book, please contact us at CustomerService@Harlequin.com.

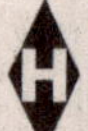

Harlequin Enterprises ULC
22 Adelaide St. West, 41st Floor
Toronto, Ontario M5H 4E3, Canada
www.Harlequin.com

HarperCollins Publishers
Macken House, 39/40 Mayor Street Upper
Dublin 1, D01 C9W8, Ireland
www.HarperCollins.com

Printed in U.S.A.

1 2 3 4 5 6 7 8 9 10 HDC 28 27 26 25

Paging Dr. Morrison

*One hospital, two doctor brothers—
and two one-night surprises!*

Mack and Rhett Morrison might look alike, might both be skilled trauma docs, and might be about to find themselves working in the same Austin ER... but that's where the similarities end. Raised by a careless father, both sons have striven to distance themselves from his influence and each other.

Mack is the steady, responsible Head of ER. Rhett has lived life on the edge as an F1 Medic, until he returns to Texas. But when a single night changes both their lives forever, the brothers must face the consequences—and fatherhood—at the same time!

In *Expecting in the ER*

Lainey has returned to Austin Memorial with shocking news for her ex-husband. Their one unplanned night of passion had consequences, and she now has a job in Mack Morrison's ER. Will the secret she's keeping tear down the walls between them, or finally tear them apart?

In *Doctor's Nine-Month Rival*

Dr. Rhett Morrison thrives on dangerous pursuits, and competing with Dr. Jacqueline Elliot for a coveted post at Austin Memorial is his toughest challenge yet! For Jacqueline turns out to be the stranger he shared one passionate night with—and she's carrying his baby!

Both available now!

Dear Reader,

My third child was a surprise baby. We love him dearly, but I can remember finding out I was pregnant and being in utter shock. All of our baby equipment had long been given away, and so we were, in essence, starting out all over again. At least we'd been through the process and knew kind of what to expect. But I was in my late thirties at the time and had some of the same fears that my character Lainey Thornton has. Plus her pregnancy comes after a sexy night in a hotel room with her ex, Mack Morrison. Let the reigniting of feelings begin!

Thank you for joining Mack and Lainey as they navigate the tricky situation of working together again and the added stress of a surprise pregnancy. They must somehow figure it out before the baby arrives, and maybe they'll find something a little extra along the way. These two characters have a special place in my heart and I found myself crying along with them at one point.

I hope you enjoy reading their story as much as I loved writing it.

Love,

Tina Beckett

Three-time Golden Heart® Award finalist **Tina Beckett** learned to pack her suitcases almost before she learned to read. Born to a military family, she has lived in the United States, Puerto Rico, Portugal and Brazil. In addition to traveling, Tina loves to cuddle with her pug, Alex; spend time with her family; and hit the trails on her horse. Learn more about Tina from her website or friend her on Facebook.

Books by Tina Beckett

Harlequin Medical Romance

Alaska Emergency Docs

Reunion with the ER Doctor

Buenos Aires Docs

ER Doc's Miracle Triplets

Jet Set Docs

Second Chance in Santiago

Sexy Surgeons in the City

New York Nights with Mr. Right

San Diego Surgeons

Expecting Her Best Friend's Baby

Resisting the Brooding Heart Surgeon
A Daddy for the Midwife's Twins?
Tempting the Off-Limits Nurse
Las Vegas Night with Her Best Friend
Nurse's Second Chance at Forever

Visit the Author Profile page
at Harlequin.com for more titles.

To my family,
who always supported me in reaching my goals!

PROLOGUE

MACK DOWNED HIS second drink of the night, mentally spent after his long day in Boston. The medical conference had been good. What hadn't been so good was spotting his ex there, today of all days, on the second anniversary of their divorce. And tomorrow he would fly home to Austin. They'd nodded at each other, but neither had moved close enough to interact or make small talk. Just as well.

She'd been upset at him for not moving from Austin when she got that job offer. Ha! Upset? Hell, thc woman had divorced him without letting him know his time to decide was up.

He thumped his glass onto the polished surface of the bar, hesitating for only a split second before raising it again as a signal that he wanted another. He wasn't driving, as his hotel was just down the street. He'd never been one to drown his sorrows, but just this once he was going to indulge himself. Everything he'd thought he wanted in life had gone up in flames, proving that lightning could indeed strike twice. First his dad. And then his wife.

You're being a damned hypocrite, Mack.

Lainey had every right to decide her future for herself. But what she didn't have a right to do was expect him to uproot himself every time she got a new job offer. Not that she'd done that. It had been just the one time. But there was no reason to think she wouldn't do it again to move a little higher on the ladder of success. Just like his dad had done—repeatedly—when he'd been a kid, leaving his boys to flounder at a new school every couple of years. It didn't matter now. It was over. And he was definitely not planning to jump into the dating pool again. Fate was evidently not going to hand him the happy, stable homelife that he'd craved as a child.

The bartender brought him the drink and put it down, sliding a folded piece of paper across the bar to him. He glanced up with a frown, and she just shrugged her shoulders with an apologetic smile. "I just do what I'm asked."

He'd already had two women proposition him tonight, and if this was what he thought it was, he was now going on three. Dammit. Just this once, couldn't he sit here and wallow in self-pity without being interrupted?

He could chuck the paper into the nearest trash, but maybe it was a phone message, which struck him as ludicrous, since he had his cell phone on him, and how would anyone even know he was at this particular bar. He flipped up the top of the note with his index finger, and it was just as he thought. There were just four words: *Look to your left*.

Before he could stop himself, his head swiveled ninety degrees, and he peered into the shadows just as someone lifted a hand that held some kind of fruity-looking drink. When his eyes tracked to her face, he froze. It couldn't be. But it was.

Had she followed him there?

No. She'd been the one who'd expected *him* to follow *her*. All the way to Boston.

Just then a song came over the bar's speakers. One that he recognized. One side of his mouth went up and he shook his head. What were the odds?

About the same as they always were for him. His smile widened. He really was wallowing in it tonight. He downed half his drink, got up from the barstool and headed over to the table where she was sitting by herself.

"Great minds, right?"

She laughed, and it was the same throaty, sexy sound that he remembered from two years ago. Although there hadn't been much laughing at the end of their marriage.

"Or stupid ones," she murmured.

There was an area of the bar that was free of tables and chairs and was evidently meant for dancing, but there was no way he was going to go out there. Not with her. Not when that song was playing. But he did pull out a chair and turn it around so that he could straddle it, setting down what remained of his drink. Then he propped his forearms on the seat's backrest. "Frozen daiquiri?"

"What else?"

He'd loved how she tasted of that particular drink when they kissed. Just the memory made him swallow. He allowed himself to smile again. "Been a long time."

Her nose crinkled, and she glanced at her watch. "Yeah, almost four hours."

This time, it was Mack who laughed. And suddenly, he knew he was going to sleep with her. He was pretty sure she was thinking the same thing, or she wouldn't have sent him that message. She would have just hunkered down in her seat in hopes that he didn't see her. Maybe she was indulging in a little pity party of her own.

He decided to test the waters. "Interested in getting out of here?"

"Is the big, bad doctor from Texas propositioning me?"

"Only if the sexy, beautiful doctor from Boston is amenable."

Her mouth twisted. "Neither of us should be driving."

"It's a good thing my hotel is just down the street then."

She took another swig of her drink and stood up, holding her hand out. "In that case…"

Wrapping his fingers around hers and getting out of his seat, he left the rest of his whiskey sitting on the table and towed her behind him. He caught the bartender's attention and threw a wad of bills on the bar, indicating it was for his and Lainey's drinks. She gave him a knowing smile.

What the bartender didn't know was that this wasn't a casual hookup. It was something just as stupid, but far more volatile. And if Mack had been in his right mind, he would never have ventured down this road. But the whiskey was whispering things to him that he couldn't seem to ignore. Things he didn't *want* to ignore. Neither he nor Lainey were making any promises. They were just going to spend a single night in each other's arms. And reminisce about how great the sex had always been between them.

And then he would fly home to Austin as if tonight had never happened…and hope that it wasn't the dumbest decision he'd ever made.

CHAPTER ONE

HOW COULD SHE have been so stupid?

Alaina Thornton wrapped one of her arms around her midsection while clutching the handle of her carry-on. It seemed she was making a lot of dumb decisions recently. Like quitting her job and packing up her apartment before she even had a new job lined up. But in all honesty, the job in Boston had been a lot more stressful than she'd thought it would be. And the idea that she could do the paperwork the position required while still practicing medicine had been a pipe dream. Her administrative role had turned into a monster that swallowed up all her time and energy and offered back nothing but headaches. She'd seen maybe six patients in the last two years. And, to her, that was not acceptable.

She had an interview at her old hospital in Austin, which she'd heard was opening up two new clinics in the city. She would love to snag a spot at either one of those. And she had purposely not called Mack for the interview, doubting that he would even give her the time of day. Especially after she'd bailed on him after their night together, choosing to sneak away at three in the morning, once she knew she was sober. She hadn't left him a note, figuring it would be the simplest thing for both of them. No long explanations about why they couldn't be together. Sleeping with him had changed nothing. Her car had been parked at the bar, so it had been easy to slip away. Too easy.

What hadn't been so easy was to forget what had happened between them.

And now…

She blew out a breath, her hand splaying over her belly. And now, she was pregnant. She'd found out two weeks ago, and had given her notice immediately afterward without giving herself time to talk herself out of it. Then she'd called the administrator at Austin Memorial and asked if there was any way she could get an interview without going through Mack, saying she was pretty much willing to take anything they had. Glenda—who'd become a good friend during her time in Austin—was the one who'd mentioned the two new clinics. She couldn't promise anything, since she said Mack was actively recruiting folks for one of the clinics, aptly named the Austin Memorial Emergency and Trauma Center, and it wouldn't be right to bypass him completely. *But*, one of the ER docs at the main hospital was retiring in a month, and she was sure that if she told Mack she had someone in mind for that position but that it had to be now, before Carter actually retired, he would be okay with it.

Lainey wasn't so sure. But her choices were pretty slim right now. She could either stay in Boston and have this baby and never mention to Mack that it was his—which was taking the easy way out, just like she'd done that night at the hotel—or she could do the hard thing and tell him the truth and let him decide what kind of role he took in their baby's life. Mack's dad had had multiple secret affairs, and there was a half sister that he'd only found out about toward the end of their marriage. He'd despised his dad, not only for cheating, but also for hiding the fact that he and his brother had a sibling.

She couldn't do that to Mack. It wasn't fair. Besides, it would come out. Eventually. Either the child would go looking for his or her dad, or Mack would find out and put two and two together and realize it was his.

Even the thought of that kind of conversation made her cringe.

The call for boarding came across the intercom, and she prayed her queasy stomach would cooperate during her flight. She was pretty sure the drinks she and Mack had consumed had affected their thinking processes, since they'd always been meticulous about birth control. At least until they'd decided to try to have a baby. It wasn't long after that that the job offer from Boston had materialized, and their relationship had imploded when he'd been unwilling to move from Austin. Well, he hadn't *said* he wouldn't. But he hadn't said that he would either.

At first she'd taken it to be a macho thing that it was always the woman who had to uproot herself to follow the man. But later, she came to understand that he simply loved his job at Austin M. But that realization hadn't changed things. She'd been determined to go, and he'd seemed just as determined to stay.

But today was the day of reckoning. She was going to have to admit to a few things: one, that her new job hadn't been all it was cracked up to be, and two, that if Mack actually *had* moved with her, he'd have been throwing away his job for nothing. Because she would have ended up leaving Boston one way or the other.

But you couldn't have known that back then.

No, but if she hadn't been so stubborn and angry, she might have dug a little deeper before jumping at the offer. Or she might have taken the job and Mack might have agreed to move with her, then when she "changed her mind" it could have still caused an irreparable split between them.

And now? Did she want to get back together with him? No. Things usually happened for a reason. Wouldn't real love have found a way to weather the storm back then?

She had no idea. One thing she did know was that she didn't want to go through the pain of breaking up all over again. And with a baby to think about, it made it even more important to weigh her options carefully. Boarding the plane and finding her seat, she decided the smartest thing she could do for all involved was to sleep—something she hadn't been able to do for the last two weeks—and hope everything would work out for the best.

Mack had to be seeing things. Glenda Silvers was standing in his ER with the very woman who spent the night with him eight weeks ago and then left without a goodbye or word of explanation. He'd woken up hours before his flight was scheduled to leave with the thought of indulging his senses one last time before they parted ways, only to discover that she'd already done the leaving.

It seemed all Lainey knew how to do was walk away without a second glance.

Well, more power to her.

So what was she doing here in Austin? With Glenda? And why was his head suddenly spinning right back toward that night in his hotel room? When those soft lips of hers had slowly worked their magic, trailing along his body's midline with aching deliberation, down, down, down, until she'd reached his…

"Can I have a word, Mack?" The administrator was now standing right in front of him, looking at him, brows drawn slightly together as if she'd somehow been party to his thoughts. Or maybe…

Hell, had Lainey somehow misconstrued things that night? Things were pretty hazy, but he knew for a fact that if she'd asked him to stop, he would have immediately called a halt to things. Had he promised her something?

No. He would remember that too. Because he hadn't been so drunk that he couldn't recall every touch. Every moan.

He took a deep breath. "Sure."

Moving to one of the walls away from anyone else, he noted that Lainey didn't come with them. Not a good sign.

"What's going on, Glenda?"

She had no problem making eye contact with

him. "You remember that Carter Jones is retiring the end of this month, right?"

"I do. I haven't started looking for that position yet. I've been kind of busy trying to finish staffing the new clinics."

"Yes. I realize that. Which is why when the perfect person came along, I didn't hesitate to scoop her up."

"The perfect person for what?" He glanced over at Lainey, who still hadn't moved. A rock settled in the pit of his stomach.

"The perfect person to replace Carter."

His teeth gritted together before he forced them apart enough to speak. "I'm the department head, Glenda. I should be making that decision."

"That's why I'm coming to you now." She gave him a hard glance. "But I will override you on this, if it becomes necessary. I have that option. I can show you where it's written in the hospital bylaws, if you need to see it."

And Glenda and Lainey were friends. He saw where this was headed. "I don't need to see it. And normally I would trust your decisions, but…" He paused. "You do know that Lainey and I are divorced, right? And that we haven't exactly been chummy over the last two years."

Except for that night in Boston. Oh, they'd been plenty chummy then.

"Yes. But that shouldn't affect your professionalism. Because Lainey has assured me that it won't affect hers. I want her back. Not just because I like her, but because she's a damned good doctor and we would be lucky to have her. *Boston* wanted her, for God's sake. They actively recruited her. The fact that she wants to come back here isn't something I'm willing to pass up. And you shouldn't either."

"Why?"

"Why what?" She tilted her head in question.

"Why does she want to come back?"

"That's for her to say, and I don't really care. But when I asked her if she was sure, she told me she was, and that's good enough for me."

Maybe it was, but it sure as hell wasn't enough for him.

But before he could say anything, she went on. "If you don't think you can work with her, then I expect you to put her in one of those new facilities. She's told me she's okay with that as well. But get one thing straight. I am hiring her, with or without your blessing."

His jaw tightened yet again. "Well, I guess there's nothing left to be said, except for me to go over and welcome her back to the team."

She gave him another hard look. "I expect you to be civil if not friendly, Mack."

"Of course." He gave a smile that held no

mirth. Yes, he could be civil. But he sure as hell wasn't going to be friendly. But he did intend to get to the bottom of this sudden change of heart of hers.

"Good." With that, Glenda gave Lainey a wave and headed toward the hallway, probably going back to her office.

Before he went over to talk to Lainey, he headed for the front desk and told them to call him if they needed him, but that he had a meeting in his office. Then he motioned to Lainey, positive that one of the nurse's mouths had dropped open. Several staff members would remember exactly who Lainey was and that they had once been married. But according to Glenda, this was a done deal. He just needed to figure out how he was going to handle working with her again. But he wasn't the type who would just tuck her away with the idea of out of sight out of mind. No. If he had to work with her, he was going to have her right here, where he could become desensitized to her presence—if that was even possible. Because he'd never become desensitized to her touch. Not during all their marriage. Not during that night in the hotel room.

But one thing he was not going to do was let himself be seduced by memories of the past.

Because some of those memories were not so good.

They got on the elevator, and he pressed the button for the second floor, which was where Mack's office was housed, and they rode up in silence. He didn't try to indulge in small talk or anything else until they reached the confines of his office, and he firmly closed the door and gestured to one of the two seats in front of his desk.

He studiously avoided looking at the pull-out couch that they had used many times, like during COVID-19 when they'd basically been shut away inside the hospital, not venturing outside of these walls. They'd made love in here on more than one occasion, and once she'd left Austin he'd barely been able to face that particular piece of furniture. And yet he couldn't bring himself to get rid of it either.

He sat behind his desk, feeling the need to keep barriers between them, including physical ones, to get the point across that they were separate beings with separate lives, despite what had happened in Boston.

"Well, it seems I am to welcome you back to the team."

"I'm sorry, Mack. I was pretty sure you would have said no, if I had come to you directly with a request to come back to work."

He nodded. "You would have guessed correctly. Which brings up the question of why you want to come back."

"Do I need a reason?"

"Frankly, yes. I'm sure it's not because I'm here."

Her teeth came down on her lower lip for a minute before she answered. "Not entirely, but it did weigh into the equation."

His brain froze, trying to process those words.

"Lainey—"

"No, stop. Before you say anything, I didn't come back in hopes that we'd get back together. That's not what either of us wants. I think we've proved that point. But there is another player in this game. One I just found out about a couple of weeks ago."

Another player?

He had no idea what she was talking about. Had Glenda asked her to come back?

"I don't understand."

She put her hands in her lap and leaned forward. "I'm pregnant, Mack."

Of all the things she might have said, this hadn't been anywhere on his radar. "Pregnant?"

His mind swept back to the night they'd spent together. Damn. He hadn't even thought about protection. It had been like muscle memory.

They hadn't used protection for months before she'd moved to Boston, because they'd wanted to have a baby. And they'd had sex in that hotel room of his…twice. It would have been more than that if she'd still been in his room the next morning. And evidently she wasn't on birth control either.

"Yes. And before you say anything, I don't want to have an abortion. I'm thirty-eight and will be close to thirty-nine when this baby is born. We both know what that means. More risks. For both the baby and for me." She blew out a breath. "This may be the only chance I get to have a child, and I want to take it."

He hadn't even thought about those risks, but now that she'd pointed them out to him, it added even more stuff for him to deal with. He and Rhett had not actually had the greatest role model when it came to fathers, and despite the fact that he and Lainey had wanted children, it had been during an idyllic period in his life when he'd been under the illusion that he could actually have dreams that came true. Well, that hadn't happened. He wasn't sure what that meant for his odds of being a halfway decent dad.

But….

He wasn't willing to say "thanks, but no thanks" either. This might be the only kid he ever had too, and by God, he wanted the opportunity to show him or her that childhood didn't have to be the shitty experience his had been. That you could actually depend on someone to be there when you needed them to be.

Like he'd been when Lainey had announced she was taking the job in Boston?

He swallowed. It was a hard truth. One he hadn't really allowed himself to dwell on. Not then. And not that night in Boston either. He hadn't been there to support her. Not physically. Not emotionally. Was she truly willing to trust him with fathering this child?

Or maybe she was just telling him all this out of courtesy. Out of the knowledge that he might someday find out.

"So I get that you want to have the baby, but what is it you want from me? Because if you tell me you don't want me involved in this child's life, I'll have to raise an objection. If it's mine—and I'm assuming you know for a fact it is, I want to be there for him or her."

"Oh it's yours." Her lips tightened. "I didn't sleep with anyone else that night."

"I didn't mean that. I just didn't know if you'd been involved with someone else."

Her eyes focused hard on his. "If I had been, it wouldn't have mattered how much I drank eight weeks ago, I wouldn't have gone back to your hotel room."

"No. Of course not." Hell, he was making a mess out of this. Just like he'd made a mess when she'd told him she had a job offer in Boston. She'd never cheated on him, and she'd never cheat on anyone else either. To have implied otherwise… He sat back in his seat. "I'm sorry, Lainey. This has just taken me by surprise."

"I know. I'm sorry too. I should have called you from Boston—before I left my job there—and told you, but I wanted to do it in person, and I'd hoped… Well, if you didn't want anything to do with the baby, I would have looked for something different. Somewhere in another part of Texas, maybe. But my mom and sisters are here, and I know they'll be excited about the baby."

So she hadn't told them yet.

He hadn't kept in touch with her family and knew that Lainey and her dad had not had the best relationship. Kind of like Mack and Thom Morrison's relationship had been. Fractious at best. Adversarial at worst.

"And your dad?"

She shrugged, and a sheen of tears appeared, but they didn't fall. "He died a year ago. Heart attack. It was sudden."

"Oh hell, Lainey, I'm sorry. I didn't know."

"It's okay. My mom didn't want a big funeral so we had a simple graveside service. It was just my sisters and me and Mom. His brother had already passed years ago, and he wasn't close with anyone else in his family."

Lainey had been in Austin a year ago and hadn't contacted him. But why would she have? They'd been divorced by that time. But there was still a sense of guilt that he hadn't known and that he hadn't sent her mom a note periodically or asked if she needed anything.

He doubted she would have wanted anything from him though. If his own mom were alive, he doubted that Lainey would have kept in contact with her either.

"I'm still sorry. I know he was a difficult person, but it still would have been hard." It brought to mind his own dad and…

Damn. That reminded him. His father had set up a trust fund for his boys and Mack's half sister. But there had been a stipulation. Mack hadn't wanted the trust fund back then and he certainly didn't want it now. Not that he had any contact with his father other than when he appeared at hospital fundraisers. But if Mack could help it, he wasn't going to tell him that Lainey was expecting a child. He did not want his dad's money, even though having a baby would have opened that up for him. So no. He was going to keep this between him and Lainey. For as long as possible.

"It was. Especially for Mom. Dad did almost everything for her and his death came out of the blue. I took her to a financial specialist, where they helped her learn the ins and outs of how to manage her money and the tax implications and how to set up automatic bill paying. It's been a big learning curve for her, but she's actually done a great job this last year. Better than Dad ever did, I think."

Maybe that's part of the reason that Lainey had such a strong sense of independence. She'd never leaned on anyone the way Marion had evidently leaned on her husband, and Mack was glad for that. He never wanted to rule over his wife or his kids. Marriage or even parenting should be a partnership with each having equal say. That it was hard to do was evident from the fact that neither he nor Lainey had been able to give in at the end of their marriage. They'd each had equal say and had ended up going their separate ways when neither had been willing to compromise. It was what it was. But he didn't regret their night together any more than he regretted their marriage. He had learned some hard lessons from the latter. But that lesson had helped keep him from making the same mistake again. With anyone.

In the two years since their marriage had ended, Mack had slept with only one woman. She'd been someone his brother, Rhett, had introduced him to at a Formula 1 race. She'd come on to him, and it was obvious that neither of them had wanted anything more than a one-night stand. He'd been very sober that night and had definitely not forgotten birth control. Neither had she. But that's all it had been: a sexual release that they hadn't felt the need to revisit. Mack hadn't gone to any more races after that, even though Rhett was the track physician at that time.

He probably should let Rhett know that he was going to be an uncle, but they hadn't exactly been close over the years. At some point he'd tell him…with the caveat that Mack didn't want their father to know.

It took him a second to remember what Lainey had just said. Something about her mom and money management. "I'm glad she's handling that okay. And that she'll be close by when you have the baby."

What did that mean for Mack? Would he have any involvement in the pregnancy part? Would he be there at the birth of their child? He didn't know the answer to any of that right now. And maybe that was okay. It would give both him and Lainey time to get their bearings and decide how to come at things.

"Me too." She stood. "Well, I should go. Glenda said I could start work sometime this week. Is that okay with you?"

This week. That was faster than he expected. "Yes. But I would like to talk to you before you start—about the job and about the baby. Is there a time we could meet? Maybe for a meal? Or even coffee at a park if you want some privacy." He smiled. "As you know, I'm not the most spontaneous person in the world. I like to plan and know what's coming so I can prepare for it."

One of her brows popped up. "Are you saying the lack of spontaneity is an always thing? Because I can definitely remember a few times when—"

He held up his hand to stop her from going any further. Because he didn't need any reminders of where or when those times had happened—he could remember every single one of them. Including the night in his motel room eight weeks ago. A night that had caused him to wake up from a sound sleep for weeks afterward. Times when he'd been hard and aching, only to look at the empty spot on the bed and remember she wasn't there. That she wouldn't be there ever again.

Well, she might not be in his bed, but it looked like the event in that hotel room was going to change the course of his life in a very permanent way. And although he was happy for Lainey.... Hell, he was happy for himself too. But it was still going to cause some complications to his life that he hadn't anticipated. And the better he could prepare for those complications, the better he would feel about the whole thing.

CHAPTER TWO

SHE AND MACK had decided to meet for lunch at one of their favorite restaurants. As soon as she mentioned the name, his face had changed and she realized she'd made a tactical error. Whereas she'd just been looking for something familiar, and Marios Trattoria and Pizzeria had come to mind, she probably should have realized it would make him uncomfortable.

He'd waved off her concerns and said it was fine. But she wasn't sure it was. And she definitely hadn't wanted to start off this new and tentative truce by making things even more strained than they already were.

He'd actually taken the news of her pregnancy better than she'd anticipated. And although part of her had expected him to refuse to have anything to do with the baby or with her, she knew that expectation hadn't been based on reality. Mack wasn't a spiteful man. But he was predictable. A tiny part of her had hoped that when she filed for divorce six months after arriving in Boston it would force his hand to either say he would relocate to be with her or say flat out that he was staying in Austin. It would have given her the yes or no answer she'd desperately needed. Instead he'd just signed the papers. But hadn't that given her her answer?

It had. But that didn't mean she'd been happy about it. And she'd missed him so badly that first year. When she'd had an awful day, he hadn't been there to hold her and make love to her and help her feel that at least one part of her life was okay. Instead, it had all been chaotic, and the hits had just kept coming. Oh, not in her career. The hospital in Boston had loved her. But unfortunately she had quickly fallen out of love with it. And then she'd seen Mack that day at the convention and had been too scared to talk to him, afraid she might pour her heart out to him. But when he happened to be at the same bar as she'd been, she suddenly needed his arms around her, even if it was all an illusion. She'd needed him to whisper to her deep in the night. To do things to her that only he could do.

And it had worked. Except once he'd fallen asleep and she lay there, staring into his face, she'd gotten this sense of panic that she'd done the wrong thing. That it was going to make her miss him all over again, undoing all of the work it had taken to live life without him. It was like she'd ripped the Band-Aid off, only to put it back on again.

She pulled into the parking lot but didn't see his car.

Then she blinked. Maybe he didn't even drive the same sporty model that he used to. She perused the cars that were there. This wasn't a cheap restaurant, and the vehicles were a reflection of that. There were a couple of black cars there, which she knew was his preference. Lainey still drove her silver Honda, a car she had a sentimental attachment to, since she'd gone to the used car lot right after getting her first paycheck as a doctor. She fell in love with her little car and put a down payment on it on the spot. Gertrude was getting up there in years now. Kind of like her, from everything she'd read in the medical journals about pregnancy.

She got out of her car, just as a familiar vehicle pulled in, parking next to her. Okay, so he hadn't gotten rid of his Beamer. She didn't know why, but that made her happy. She had a lot of good memories of riding in that car. Of doing other things in that car. Things that had made her heart quicken and her body come alive.

Mack came from money, but he'd always

been determined to make his own way in this world. He didn't want to rely on his dad for anything…never asked the man for anything. And she'd respected him for that. In some ways they were alike. Her father had been the unchallenged head of the household, at least until Lainey, the youngest, came along. She understood that he felt the family needed a leader, but it was an unhealthy codependent kind of leadership where he ruled over everything with a fist of iron. Lainey was the only one to openly defy him—even her sisters didn't do that.

Mack's dad was wealthy and expected people to jump at his every whim. Even his boys. And his wife—who died when his sons were just coming into adulthood. His second wife was almost a carbon copy of his first.

Like Lainey, Mack chafed against the limits his dad placed on everything. It was part of what had drawn her to him. She thought he'd be the one person to understand her. And then came Boston, proving her wrong.

Mack joined her on the sidewalk. "Ready?"

"Yes, thanks for agreeing to come here. I couldn't think of anything else when you mentioned going out to eat."

"It's fine. I've been here plenty of times since we…"

Since they'd split. She got it. But immediately that thought was replaced with wondering if he'd brought other women here. She quickly squashed the notion. Well, as best she could.

"I get it. Hopefully the place hasn't changed too much."

"It's still run by the same family, so no. It hasn't." He smiled. "They still serve your favorite dish."

"Mmm, the ravioli Fiorentina?"

"Yep."

She wasn't surprised that he remembered that, since she almost always ordered that dish, despite perusing the menu each and every time. But in her head, nothing could compete with the ravioli. Mack, surprisingly, was much more adventurous in trying new things from the menu. She would expect him to be the one who always wanted the same thing. Mack hated change. He wanted things to be predictable. Comfortable. She understood why he didn't want to move with her to Boston, but in reality, life was never going to be predictable or comfortable. And sometimes you had to be willing to make changes or you became stagnant.

She shook off the memories, because they did nothing but make her brood about things that couldn't be changed.

They were quickly shown to a table, and the hostess—a cute blonde who had to be at the low end of her twenties—greeted Mack by name. To Mack's credit, although he smiled at her, he didn't flirt or give her anything more than a friendly hello back.

Lainey quickly buried her head in her menu, and when she chanced a glance over the top of it, she found Mack with his eyes on her. "What?"

"Nothing."

But it didn't seem like nothing. Was he regretting her telling him she was pregnant? He'd seemed shocked, but he'd also seemed certain of wanting to play a role in the baby's life. But that would also mean that whole life change thing she'd thought about earlier. So maybe he was rethinking that.

She put down her menu. "Seriously. If you want to just talk about work and worry about the rest…later…we can."

"By 'the rest' I assume you're referring to the baby."

"I am."

He took a deep breath and let it come out in an audible sigh. "No, I thought about that a lot last night, and to ignore the fact that I'm going to be a parent doesn't sit well with me. Nor does letting you do all of this by yourself."

But he said nothing about what he wanted.

"I'm a big girl. And people parent on their

own all the time. I'm well aware that you didn't choose this. Nor did you have any say in whether or not I let the pregnancy go to term. But you do have a choice about whether you want to be a part of the child's life. What do you want to do, Mack? I will be okay, I promise. I can walk this journey on my own. And honestly it would be a whole lot less complicated if I'm the only one who..."

She stopped herself before the words she'd been thinking came out. But it was true. It would be a lot easier if she were the only one calling the shots. Because she'd seen for herself that she and Mack could very easily wind up on opposite sides of the spectrum when it came to making decisions about the future.

He frowned. "Do you not want me involved? Why come back if that's the case?"

The waiter came to the table and took their orders before she could think of an answer. And the truth was she had thought about staying away. But she knew she owed it to Mack to tell him the truth. That had always been important to her. Though she'd always just blurted out her truth without thinking much about how she said things. When she'd chosen to go to Boston, she'd made the decision and immediately told Mack without any foreplay or more subtle lead up to the news. She'd done the same thing about the pregnancy. The first day she was back, she just spewed the news and expected him to decide one way or the other.

She tried to backtrack, but that was not her forte either. Her tendency was to keep on pushing forward to whatever goal she had in mind. And right now the goal was to have this baby and have a plan of action in place.

Once they had their drinks though, she made an attempt. "I wanted you to have a choice one way or the other. There's still time for you to think it through. But I would like to have an answer sometime before the baby is born."

His head tilted. "I already gave you my answer. And I don't go back on my word."

This was not going well. It felt like the path they'd traversed once before. The one that had led to their divorce. "I know you don't. But please give yourself some time and space to decide what kind of role you want to play."

A muscle worked in his jaw, and he took a drink of his water before answering. "How much time, exactly, do I have? One month? Or maybe you'd prefer six? I'd like to know before it becomes too late."

She'd asked for the divorce six months after she moved to Boston, and that was probably a mistake. She should have come back and tried to engage him in a conversation about it. But she had been hurt and felt like if he wanted to be with her, he would have moved. Only Mack knew whether or not that had been the truth. They'd both made mistakes during that process. But this time, another life was involved, and she wanted things spelled out as clearly as possible. She wanted to be proactive rather than reactive.

"Tell me how much time you think you'll need."

He leaned forward. "Lainey, I've already told you. I want to be involved in this child's…in *my* child's life. And that won't just involve writing a monthly check."

Is that what he thought she wanted? Money? "I make a very good living, thank you very much. I don't need your money."

There was a standoff as they eyed each other—like enemies who were sizing up their opponent.

She held up a hand before he could react to her words. "Mack, just this once, can we move to the same side of the field and play on the same team? We may not be married anymore, but for this to work, we have to be able to agree on things, no matter how we feel about each other."

"Understood. I'll try."

The problem was, she wasn't sure how she

felt about him. Coming back here had caused a strange medley of emotions to play across her heart. But she smiled just as their plated food was placed in front of them before saying, “So will I. Now, shall we eat and talk about something else? Tell me how the ER is doing at Austin M and what kind of changes there have been.”

They talked shop in between bites, and not surprisingly, there had been very little change to the program other than a few new pieces of equipment and some new staff members. Mack was a good leader and the turnover rate in the department was one of the lowest at the hospital. If the offer from Boston hadn’t come in, she would have probably stayed too, and not just because she’d been married to the department head.

And they would probably still be married. And maybe already have a child of their own.

A jolt to her system had her closing her eycs for a second or two.

But if a job offer had been all it took to tear them apart, something else probably would have come along later and caused a division.

And sleeping with him after the convention? A moment of weakness on her part. One that wouldn’t be repeated. Couldn’t be repeated, for her own sanity. Maybe she should find out exactly how closely she'd be working with him. After all, everyone that knew them before she left would wonder why she was back and whether she and Mack were getting back together. And soon enough, her pregnancy was going to be evident. But she would tackle all of that when it came.

"Thanks for the update. Where do you see me fitting in? At the main hospital? At one of the new clinics? Will they both have some kind of ER capability?"

"One of them will be a mini-ER/trauma center. We've always had a problem with having more patients than available beds at Austin Memorial. Hopefully this will take some of the strain off the main hospital and it will help us reach those in the community that might not otherwise make the trip to our ER. The cases that for whatever reason can't be handled there, will be transported here. There's a dedicated medical transport system that will operate between the two facilities."

She nodded. That made sense. "And the other clinic?"

"It is actually called Austin Memorial Family Birth Center. It offers state-of-the-art care for maternity patients. It has an operating room that can handle C-sections and other surgeries and will also have a variety of natural options that our patients might prefer, like midwife care and birthing pools. It's still relatively new, but there's already a lot of interest."

She sat up straighter. Lainey had been doing a lot of thinking about where she might want to have this baby, and this might be the perfect option. She knew the staff at Austin Memorial and trusted them to provide the best care. There would be an expectation of the same high-quality treatment at any new facility they opened. "Are they accepting patients yet?"

"Yes, they just started. Are you thinking of going there for prenatal care? We still have a maternity ward at Austin M, but we'll be phasing that out and sending more and more of our patients to the new clinic. Again, it will help with the shortage-of-bed issues. We will probably keep maternity patients who are dealing with multiple issues that would impact their pregnancies, like known cardiac problems, insulin resistance, etcetera."

"That makes sense. And yes, I might consider going there. It would be easier, don't you think? It'll give us some more privacy during the process. I'd already been thinking along those lines. I know we won't be able to keep the pregnancy a secret, but I'd rather not be seen at Austin M."

It was funny how easily the hospital's nickname still rolled off her tongue after two years. And how heartbreakingly familiar it was to look into Mack's eyes, or the way his smile had always pierced her armor with such ease. It still did that, as evidenced by their night together.

She'd remembered each and every inch of Mack's body on that fateful night, and had known exactly what to do to bring him the most pleasure. And he'd remembered her special spots. Oh how he'd remembered…

Mack was talking, and she struggled to tune back in, but finally realized he was giving her the names of some other clinics, if she wanted to go completely out of Austin Memorial's network. "I'm sure the administration will understand if you go to one of our competitors."

His grin sent a sharp pain through her midsection, giving evidence to her earlier thoughts. This man knew just how to get to her, without even trying.

Not for the first time, she wondered if it was a good idea to come back to the hospital. Maybe she hadn't learned her lesson after that quick decision to leave Austin two years ago. Because it seemed her more recent move home had been just as speedy. Maybe she should clear things up.

"Mack, what happened in Boston…well, it can't happen again. It brings back too many painful memories." She gave a shrug. "I'm sorry."

"I never assumed it would. And I happen to agree with you. I'm not interested in the whole friends with benefits mentality either."

Was he saying they were still friends? After everything that had happened? It sure didn't feel like it right now, but she hoped that maybe… just maybe they could get back to that. Because she sure could use a friend. She still had to tell her mom about the pregnancy and somehow explain to her that while she and Mack would be co-parenting this child, that's all they would be doing. Her mother had loved Mack like a son, and it was no wonder. He had always treated Lainey with respect. A respect that her mother had lacked during her own marriage.

"I'm not interested in that either. But I'm not sorry about the pregnancy."

He reached across the table and squeezed her hand. "I know you're not. And I'm happy for you, Lainey." There was a slight pause. "Happy for both of us."

But was he really? That hesitation made her wonder. Maybe she was reading too much into it. But men didn't have the same time constraints that women did. It wasn't fair, but it was reality. Someday Mack might find love again and start a family with his new partner.

What would that mean for their own baby through the years? If she knew Mack, it wouldn't change how he felt about this child. Like he said, he always kept his word. He wouldn't show favoritism except to whoever his new wife was. But then again, Lainey didn't plan to ask a lot of Mack. Just that his presence in his child's life remain steady. She wouldn't put up with months of sporadic contact. He was either in or he was out, which was why she'd wanted him to take some time to think about what he was going to do and then stick to whatever he decided.

They'd both finished their meals and had waved away the wait staff when they asked about dessert or coffee. Lainey couldn't eat another bite, and she was trying to monitor her caffeine intake. But they couldn't both sit here forever either, even though she wasn't quite ready to leave. But maybe she could do something else instead.

"Is there a chance I can see the new clinics? Especially the new ER building, if you decide that's where you want me?"

"Sure. We've put out some job notices on that one to get the staff levels up to where they need to be. And since you have administrative experience now, you might want to apply for head of—"

"No."

He leaned back. “Excuse me?”

She realized how that must have sounded. “The administrative stuff was why I ended up leaving Boston.” She tried to think about how to put it other than to flat out say that she’d made a mistake by going. “I realized I loved the medicine side of things a whole lot more than I did the constant putting out of fires in the department, whether it was squabbles between doctors or issues between the board and staff. I came here to get away from that.”

“And here I thought you came back for me.”

She froze until he shook his head and added, “I’m kidding, Lainey.”

“Oh.” What else could she say? She felt somewhat deflated by the way his words made her shift her expectations about friendship and whether or not things between them could improve enough to actually benefit their child.

Could they? There had been so many hard feelings between them, was it even something they could overcome? And if not, what would a toxic relationship do to her pregnancy and to the baby?

“When do you want to take a look at the clinics? I do have to be back at the hospital for a few hours today, and Rhett called me out of the blue and wants to talk.”

That surprised Lainey. Mack and his brother's relationship had always been… Strained was probably the best way to put it. "Are you guys talking again?"

"Not as often as we probably should. I think something may have happened at the track that he wants to discuss."

She knew Rhett had been a physician at one of the big F1 racetracks and that he himself had been involved in racing, something Mack had never really approved of. Lainey thought it was more worry than anything, which she could understand. But he and his brother had had a couple of tense discussions over the phone when she and Mack were still married. It was just a case of two brothers with very different personalities and different goals in life. Hopefully they could someday settle into a relationship that wasn't filled with conflict.

She blinked. Maybe it was like her and Mack. They had different personalities…different goals…and the end of their marriage had been filled with conflict.

Surely if there was hope for peace between Mack and his brother, there was hope for her and her ex-husband.

At least that was her prayer.

"It doesn't have to be today. I actually need to go with my mom to look for an apartment to rent. She wants me to stay with her, but…"

“I get it. Okay, so not this afternoon, and I have a full day tomorrow, but how about on Wednesday? I have the day off.”

“That sounds perfect. Maybe by then I’ll have moved my stuff into my new place and can wrap my head around all the changes that are taking place in my life.”

She was pretty sure Mack needed some time to do the same thing, so having a day or two to let things sink in would probably help both of them. Then they could come back together and, between the two of them, figure some things out.

And if they couldn’t?

Then she’d better hope the new ER clinic had a place for her, because she didn’t see herself being able to work with Mack on a day-to-day basis, no matter what she’d hoped for when she left Boston.

CHAPTER THREE

MONDAY AFTERNOON AND Tuesday had been tough days for Mack, and he hadn't had much time for any kind of deep introspection. Rhett had had a crisis at his job and was thinking about making a change. What kind of change was yet to be seen.

And yesterday, there'd been a multi-vehicle collision on I-35 due to heavy fog. The visibility had also impeded first responders who were trying to get to those injured. Austin M had ended up taking four critical patients, two of which were still in intensive care with life-threatening injuries.

And today he had to meet Lainey. And discuss their future. As if he had any answers. Their lunch meeting had been tense. And adding to the tension had been those familiar little gestures that he remembered far too well. The way she tucked her dark hair behind her ears when she ate, exposing those dainty earlobes that he'd loved to kiss. The way she would pause with her fork halfway to her mouth when she was intently listening to what the other person was saying. She'd done that several times when he'd been talking.

It had always made him feel important, and yesterday was no different. It was as if she was putting everything on pause so that she didn't miss any part of what he was saying. And it still made him feel just as special as it used to. Only this time there was an ache in his chest. Because it wasn't the reality of the situation. He was no longer part of her life. At least not as a romantic partner. So her listening skills had nothing to do with him. It was simply her way of conversing. He needed to remember that, or he was going to find himself in another situation like the one that happened at the hotel.

So how was he going to ignore those remembered nuances that made Lainey who she was—that had always made him want her with a fervor that had been unmatched?

And to sit in a car with her and go on a tour of the new clinics? Where he was hyperaware of everything she did—hyperaware of her scent as it drifted past him. But what choice did he have? He'd told her he would take her.

Right now, though, he just felt wrung out.

But he'd better pull himself together. Because he was due to meet her in the hospital parking lot in fifteen minutes. He guessed he should be thankful she hadn't asked him to pick her up in front of her mother's house. Because he couldn't think of anything more awkward than that: to have to make small talk with Marion Thornton while Lainey shifted from foot to foot looking miserable.

Had she even told her mom she was pregnant?

He had no idea. But maybe he'd better ask. Because it wasn't only her mom he needed to think about—it was her three older sisters, who'd already raised their children, the youngest of which was probably just getting ready to graduate from high school, if he remembered their ages correctly.

He turned into the hospital's lot with ten minutes to spare and found Lainey already there, sitting on one of the benches in front of the building, the peaked entry of the four-story edifice seeming to tower over her.

Pulling up in front of her, he leaned over and opened the door. "You're early."

"Does that surprise you?" She got into the car and closed the door behind her.

He waited until she'd fastened her seat belt

before heading away from Austin M. “No. You always were punctual.”

And there was that scent. Right on cue. A mix of warm vanilla and everything Lainey. Sexy as hell. He swallowed, trying to somehow banish it from his system. But it was proving to be a losing battle.

“I guess that’s one way we’re alike,” she said. “You never tended to run late either. It was more of a race to see who could arrive the earliest.”

He laughed. “You normally did land on top.”

“You never seemed to mind me being on top when we were married.” Her hand came up to cover her mouth, eyes wide and horrified looking. “I have no idea why I said that. Ignore that comment.”

How could he ignore something that brought an excruciatingly vivid image to mind? Of Lainey straddling his hips, her head thrown back as she slowly rose and fell, her body molding tightly around his.

Oh hell. His body wasn’t taking those memories lying down either. It had begun to rise to the occasion in the most uncomfortable way.

“Consider it ignored.” And that was lie number one of the day. And it had happened less than thirty seconds after she’d climbed into his car. How many more would there be before the day ended?

She cleared her throat. "Did you hear about that accident on the highway yesterday morning?"

"We actually got several patients from that accident."

"Oh that's right. We always did have a great trauma center."

"We still do."

Lainey turned to look at him, chin raised. "I didn't mean to imply otherwise."

The words were crisp and formal and told him exactly where he stood: on the outside looking in.

"I know."

And just like that, his body was back under control. It looked like this was how it was going to be again, with each of them being overly sensitive to comments made by the other. And having to be quick to reassure that that's not what they had meant.

Vestiges of the way their marriage had crumbled and died. But hopefully they could find their way to solid ground and stay there rather than returning to the mire over and over.

He decided to change the subject. "Did you get a chance to tell your family about the baby?"

"I told my mom last night. But I still need to tell my sisters. Mom is over the moon. This baby will be her fifteenth grandchild."

"I remember all of those nieces and nephews. We had them over more than a few times."

Lainey smiled, and it lit up her face. "They always did love their Uncle Mack."

That was the hard thing about divorce. It wasn't just the loss of a marriage, but the loss of an extended family. He had loved those kids just as much as they'd loved him. They'd grown up around him. And he'd made no effort to keep up with any of them.

How could he have? There wasn't really an instruction manual on how to dissolve all of those relationships.

"Your sisters are great."

"We have a good relationship now. But when we were growing up…not so much. I'm sure they all thought I was a bratty little kid who didn't want to do anything I was told."

This was another area where he and Lainey truly were alike. Neither of them had gotten along well with their fathers. For different reasons, and as far as he knew, Lainey's dad had never cheated on his wife, but he'd been kind of a bully, nonetheless. Mack had always felt the need to protect Lainey from him, but Lainey wouldn't have it. She didn't need protection and proved it on many occasions. She could stand up for herself quite well when the need arose.

Kind of like she'd stood up to him when Mack asked her to stop and take a breath about the offer from Boston. As soon as he'd said the words though, he knew it was the wrong thing to say to her. She just dug her heels in and made her decision within days.

Mack's rudder couldn't keep up with hers. Where she could pivot and shift directions at a moment's notice, he needed time to study whatever situation was at hand and then slowly turn angle by angle, foot by foot.

"You just always knew what you wanted and no one was going to stand in your way."

He hadn't meant it as a cut nor was he referring to her decision to leave Boston, but from the change in her face, he could tell that's the way she took it.

"Maybe we should skip the visit to the clinics."

He pulled into the nearest parking lot, which happened to be one of the big-box stores, and stopped at a random spot. Then he turned and touched her cheek. "I'm sorry, Lainey. I wasn't talking about Boston, I swear. I was referring to how you stood up to your dad. I always admired that about you. Your mom and your sisters just did whatever he wanted you guys to do. I know he's gone and I shouldn't be speaking ill of the dead, but it's true."

Her face softened and she nodded. "Yes it was. And despite the fact that I'll always love him, I also didn't want to become my mom, letting people walk all over me." Her mouth twisted and she leaned into his hand. "I think I expected people to do that, even you. But it wasn't true. You never made me feel like that."

He couldn't stop his thumb from brushing across the warm skin beneath his touch. It was every bit as silky and soft as he remembered.

"Maybe because I know what it feels like to not have control over what happens in your life. My dad was similar to yours in a lot of ways."

"I think so too. Maybe that's why we butted heads sometimes."

"Agreed." He let his hand drop before the moment grew more intimate. He needed to be careful this didn't head into territory that would be hard to come back from. "Are you still okay with going? Or would you rather go back to the hospital?"

"I'd like to see the clinics, if possible."

"Of course. I'm anxious for you to see them."

And that was true. He was proud of what Austin M had accomplished since she'd been gone. How many times had he wished he could call her and tell her about something or other that had happened at the hospital? Lots and lots. But of course he couldn't.

They pulled back into traffic and were able to find some lighter topics to discuss. "So did I tell you I participated in the Boston Marathon last year and fell flat on my face within sight of the finish line?" she asked.

"You didn't! Did you get hurt?"

"No, but I was embarrassed. Someone once said you know you're old when instead of laughing when you fall, people all run up to offer assistance."

"You're not old, Lainey."

She was still the most beautiful woman he'd ever laid eyes on. In fact, she just seemed to get better with every year that passed.

"Tell that to my future obstetrician. I'm pretty sure he or she will disagree with you."

"I'm pretty sure I'll have to disagree with that doctor."

She laughed again. "When I'm nine months pregnant, I'll probably be in full agreement with them. I don't think any of my sisters had children when they were my age. They all started their families when they were much younger."

"It doesn't matter what they did. This is your baby. Your decision. And that includes timing."

"I'm sure medical school had something to

do with that. I waited longer than I might've waited otherwise."

They were nearing the Austin Memorial Emergency and Trauma Center, and Mack turned into the entrance just off a tree-lined street. Parking was on the opposite side of the building, as was the ambulance bay. He found a shady spot and pulled in. He decided to change the subject. "This is clinic number one."

Lainey got out at the same time as he did and shut the door. "Wow. It looks like a mini version of Austin M."

With an entry that reminded him of the bow of a boat, coming together at a sharp angle in front, they'd purposely constructed the clinics to look cohesive. Just smaller. They were both single-story buildings, whereas the main hospital was four stories tall.

"Yes, the board wanted them to be recognizable as part of the Austin Memorial hospital system."

"Well, they sure accomplished that," she said. "Do I know anyone who works here?"

"I don't think so. We're trying to staff them with new folks rather than pull them from Austin M. The fear was that our house staff might try to compare the clinic to the main hospital campus, when there needs to be two different mindsets."

"And yet I worked at the main campus. Does that knock me out of the running for working here?"

"No. It's been two years since you worked at Austin M. But your hospital in Boston was a behemoth facility. These clinics are going to seem tiny by comparison."

She stopped and eyed the facade of the building. "I think that might be appealing at this point. It might not seem quite as overwhelming as Boston was. In more ways than one."

He could see that. "Ready to go in? These are both still works in progress. They've only been up a few months. As word of mouth spreads about the new centers, the hope is that they'll become much busier. Which is why we've been actively recruiting new staff for both places."

"Do you already have a lot of applications coming in?"

"Not as many as you might think. There's been a shortage of emergency care and trauma docs in the area—probably in the country, actually. So we work hard to keep what we have."

Lainey gave him a quick look.

Did she think he didn't try hard enough to keep what he had? *Who* he had? Looking back at it, she was probably right. But when two people's goals no longer aligned, wasn't it time to throw in the towel? Or had Mack taken the easy way out?

If that was true of him, then it applied to Lainey too. Neither of them had seemed very interested in fighting for their marriage. Of course that was hard to do from different sides of the country. And from opposite sides of the line of scrimmage.

Rather than trying to respond, he opened the front door to let her go into the building.

There were several people in the waiting room, and it was louder than you expected it to be from its serene exterior. Most emergency rooms were that way though. One of the staff members who wasn't busy signing someone in waved him over. "Hi, Dr. Morrison. You're bringing us some help, I hope?"

"Are you swamped?"

"I wouldn't say swamped, but give us a few more months and we'll start feeling the pinch. Right now we can keep up. Being good at what we do is a double-edged sword. Word of mouth spreads fast."

"Don't I know it. We're doing our best to get you some help. If you know of anyone, please send them my way."

"I will."

He gestured toward Lainey. "This is Lainey…" He realized he wasn't sure how to introduce her.

"I'm Lainey Thornton. I'm an ER doc who's just moving back to the area."

Ah…so she'd gone from being Lainey Thornton-Morrison to being just Lainey Thornton again. He wasn't sure why that stung, but it did. It was like she'd erased his presence in her life.

Hell, Mack, isn't that what divorce is all about?

He didn't have time to dissect the ins and outs of that phrase because Sofie was busy telling Lainey how great things were at the clinic and how thrilled they'd be if she came to work there.

"We're not sure where Lainey is going to wind up. I'm just showing her both new clinics today."

Sofie crinkled her nose. "Well, keep us in mind if you're given the option, please."

"I will."

Mack motioned toward the door leading to the back of the clinic. "I'm going to show her around, okay?"

"Sure. It was nice meeting you, Dr. Thornton."

"Call me Lainey, please." She smiled at Sofie before following him through the door.

Once they arrived in the exam room area, it looked like a normal emergency room. Mack watched as she perused the space. “How many beds do you have?”

“Right now we have ten, but we purposely built larger than we needed, so we can double our capacity as our patient load grows.”

“How many more doctors are you looking to hire?”

“Two right now. But again, as the need grows so will our staff.”

She smiled at him. “Congratulations, this is great. How did you fund it?”

“Actually, an anonymous donor stepped up and paid for both the facilities.”

“Completely?”

“Yep.” He knew what she was going to ask before she opened her mouth. “I have no idea who it was, and I doubt Glenda does either. From what I understand, the person did not want it made public.”

“Wow,” she said. “Most people would want it shouted from the rooftops.”

“Evidently not this person. And maybe it’s better that we don’t know.” Mack had wondered a couple of times if his father could have had a hand in the opening of these facilities, but he normally liked the attention. Liked having things named after him. But what if this time he didn’t?

Would he love these clinics as much if Thom Morrison had had them built?

As much as he hated to admit it, he probably wouldn't, and Mack wasn't sure why that was, other than the fact that his father rarely gave anything without attaching one or more strings to the gift. Which was another reason he didn't think it was his dad. And Rhett had never mentioned the clinics either. Although why he thought his brother would know when Mack didn't…

He made quick work of showing her around, pleased more than he should have been by Lainey's seeming excitement over different little things in the place. Like a small but mighty coffee shop that had an actual barista and a decent selection of specialty coffee drinks. She went in and ordered a decaf latte with blackberry, lavender and white chocolate syrup.

When Mack made a face, she laughed. "I know. But a colleague in Boston brought one in and let me try it, and I was hooked. Except I'm drinking decaffeinated nowadays."

The barista handed her the drink, and she took a sip, then offered the cup to Max. He shook his head. "Lavender is not a food.

"I beg to differ. Look it up."

"Okay, I'll change my answer to 'lavender is not a food I want to partake of.'"

He was kind of being ridiculous, but the thought of drinking from the same spot that Lainey's lips had just touched made him uneasy. Maybe because they had been so quick to share food and drinks while they'd been married. It had been a comfortable, intimate thing that neither had thought twice about doing. But not anymore. Despite their night in Boston, their relationship wasn't comfortable or intimate. And to try to get back to that point was to put himself in danger of being hurt again. Or left behind. Again. And neither of those options was acceptable.

It was better to just live and let live. Lainey could do her thing and he would do his.

And after the baby was born?

He had no idea.

"Ready to go to the other clinic?" he asked.

She glanced at her watch. "Yikes, I didn't realize that much time had gone by. I'm supposed to go sign the lease on my new apartment in two hours. Do you mind if I see it another time? Or I can come by myself, if I'll be working at the main facility instead of one of the clinics. Does the birth center have an ER section as well?"

"It does, but since most of those patients are maternity, it's staffed as such."

He was slightly disappointed that she couldn't

go to the birth center today, but then again, maybe it was for the best. Maybe, like she'd said earlier, he did need a little more time to adjust to the reality of the pregnancy. "I think Glenda has taken the choice of where you'll be working out of my hands."

And despite what he'd thought earlier, he wasn't sure he would say no if she asked him today about rejoining the Austin Memorial team. Yet three days ago, he wouldn't have hesitated to veto her return. Maybe he was more amenable to the idea because he had no choice. Or maybe it was just that she'd shown that they could actually get along—somewhat. At least today they could. Who knew about tomorrow.

But Mack hoped this was the start of something that wouldn't leave him bitter and angry the way the divorce had. It wasn't so much that he could see things from Lainey's point of view now as they'd gotten past hurling words at each other that neither of them meant.

That was a good sign, wasn't it?

Only time would tell. But he could hope.

CHAPTER FOUR

"GRAB SOME GLOVES, plastic dressings and tape, and meet me at the café."

Mack's hurled words gave her a burst of adrenaline that counteracted the exhausting shift she'd just lived through. Her first day at work had certainly been eventful. She'd seen ten patients over the course of five hours, and she still had three more hours to go until she could settle into a warm tub. No hot baths for her. At least not for the next several months.

She and Mack had been scheduled for the same shift, and whether that was on purpose or just a fluke, she had no idea. As the department head, he didn't need to be on the floor as much as the other doctors and staff, but she knew from their time together that he would put in his hours and then do his paperwork on his own time. If she could have done that in Boston maybe life there wouldn't have seemed as much like clocking in and out of any corporate-type job. But that hadn't been an option. She'd been expected to be in her office—and accessible to anyone who might want to drop in to chat or had a question—a certain number of hours every day, although she normally had weekends off.

If she thought this was physically grueling, Boston had sucked her dry of any mental or emotional energy. She'd take physical tiredness any day of the week.

Supplies in hand, she sprinted in the direction of the café, muscle memory from over two years ago guiding her steps.

She heard the commotion before she arrived. Several people were standing outside the café, a couple of them looking ill. What on earth had happened?

Ducking through the door, she didn't see anyone immediately. "Mack?"

"Back here."

His voice came from behind the counter, somewhere out of sight.

She hurried toward him and found him crouched beside the café's manager, who Lainey remembered from her time here. There was blood everywhere.

Maria saw her and tried to smile. "I—I wasn't even running with them."

Just then, Lainey saw the handles of a pair

of scissors sticking out of the woman's upper right quadrant. She handed Mack the kit she'd brought then quickly washed her hands in the sink and pulled on the gloves. "I believe you. But let's get you patched up."

Just then a strange wet sucking sound came from under the woman's shirt. Lainey's eyes jerked up and Mack nodded.

"Let's cut her clothing away from the scissors as much as possible."

While Lainey worked on that, Mack got out what he needed, including the medical plastic and tape and laid them out on a sterile drape he'd spread over the floor.

The scissors had evidently punctured one of Maria's lungs, and air was being dragged in and out through the opening in her chest every time she took a breath. "How do you want to seal it?"

She wasn't asking for the technique, since she knew how to close a sucking chest wound to keep air from building up in the cavity—which would make it harder and harder for Maria to breathe. If the scissors weren't there, they would simply cover the wound with gauze and tape it on three sides. It would allow trapped air to escape but seal the opening with each inhale and prevent any more from entering her chest. But the scissors were in their way, and to remove them without knowing exactly what structures the blades were near could mean nicking the pulmonary artery or other vessels. Surgery was the only way to make sure that didn't happen.

"We'll cut a slit through one side of the plastic and lay it around the blades, taping it in place, and then do the three sides like we normally would."

She swallowed. Even wiggling the blades could spell danger. But there was no other option. "Do you have a surgeon on the way?"

"Yes. He's just finishing up a procedure."

While Mack prepared to do what he needed to, his movements confident and methodical, Lainey decided to explain to Maria what their plan was. Knowledge was power and would help to keep the woman calm. At least she hoped so. "We're not going to take the scissors out. Dr. Morrison is going to close your wound until a surgeon can take a look at you, okay? One is on his way down."

The woman nodded. "But what about the café? We're shorthanded today and—"

"Don't worry about that. I'll stay here until we can find someone to take over."

She saw Mack's frown even as he slid the plastic into place on either side of the scissors. She didn't care. The last thing Maria needed to worry about was her establishment sitting empty in her absence.

Mack readied the tape. "Okay, Maria, I need you to exhale as much as possible and hold it for a minute."

She did as instructed, groaning in pain as her chest deflated. Lainey's ex was quick though and had the tape in place within seconds. He touched her shoulder, "Okay, go ahead and breathe normally."

Maria did as he asked.

"Better?" Lainey held her breath, hoping Mack's plan had worked. It was the normal protocol for sealing a chest wound with an object still in place, but there was always the fear that it wouldn't work or that the patient would go on to develop a pneumothorax, where air became trapped in the chest cavity. It was why they only sealed three sides of the plastic and left the fourth open. The hope was that any air that gathered would escape through the opening.

Just then an orderly arrived with a gurney and one of the nurses, followed by a tall, thin man who Lainey assumed was the surgeon. She didn't recognize him though.

He knelt down. "Ah, no need to ask what happened to you. I'm Dr. Jefferson, one of Austin M's thoracic surgeons. We're going to take you up to surgery and get those scissors removed, okay?"

"Can you let my daughter know where I am?"

"We will." He motioned to the nurse, who had a tablet and got the daughter's name and phone number, and Maria, to her credit, was able to sign and authorize surgery, despite the pain she must be in.

Between the team, they got her lifted onto the gurney. As they were getting ready to leave, Maria grabbed her hand. "You'll stay at the café until my daughter gets here? She knows how to run everything."

Lainey had just assumed that the woman wanted her daughter there, in case something happened during surgery, but leave it to Maria to worry first about her café and then about herself. "I'll wait here, don't you worry."

Then they were off. Mack turned to her. "You don't have to wait. We can just close the café doors and put up a sign."

"No. I promised. Besides, it'll give me a chance to get the blood cleaned up. Maria's daughter shouldn't have to come in to that."

Mack looked at her and then touched her hand. "You always were a softy."

The warmth of his hand threatened to turn her insides to mush, but she couldn't seem to turn away.

"I just want to do the right thing, and in this case, it feels right." She paused. "If things get busy in the ER they can call me."

"I'll stay and help."

She smiled at him and then squeezed his hand. When a wave of emotion came out of the blue and threatened to swamp her, she let go of him and turned away. Where had that come from?

It had to be pregnancy hormones. At least she wasn't sick today. But it was a reminder that she did need to make an appointment to be seen at the clinic. She hadn't even thought about what kind of birth experience she wanted and wasn't actually sure they would give her the option due to her age.

And if they felt she was too high-risk to take on?

Then she'd have to find another hospital, even if it was one of the competitors' facilities like Mack had joked. If Maria had recognized her, there were undoubtedly countless other people here who would too. And the last thing she wanted was to answer the samc questions over and over. And surely Mack didn't want to have to deal with that either.

While he went to shut the door and put up the closed sign, she went to work, cleaning up their triage area, gathering the bloody gauze and so forth into a plastic bag that she would later put into one of the hazardous waste bins.

Mack came back with some disinfectant, and

they wiped everything down that had—or possibly *could* have—come into contact with any bodily fluids. Then they discarded the veggies that Maria had been chopping on a plastic cutting board and loaded it into the industrial dishwasher.

"She must have been using the scissors to cut open the bag of lettuce and somehow fallen," she said.

"I was thinking the same thing." He pulled down two cups. "Do you want a coffee?"

"I would love one. Decaf for me though. Do you know how to work the espresso machine?"

His brows went up and she laughed. "Of course you do. I almost forgot that we had one of those at home."

Home. Even saying that word made her throat clog.

Although how could she have forgotten about the espresso machine? How many times had Mack brought her a cup of coffee in bed as part of their morning ritual? Sometimes that cup gave her a much-needed jolt of energy and sometimes it was abandoned for another—more sensual—type of pick-me-up.

And there was that emotional wave again. Damn. She was going to have to figure out how to deal with the memories that were going to be inevitable since she would be seeing the man on a regular basis.

She watched as he set down the demitasse cups and filled and tamped coffee into the double-sided portafilter before he tightened it onto the machine. Then he pressed start. The machine hissed and sputtered, and finally the scent of coffee tickled her nose as the pressurized stream of the dark brew trickled into the cups under the spouts. Then he rinsed out the filter and set it on a towel to dry.

They went over to one of the bar-height tables and sat down. Lainey took a packet of sugar and dumped it into her espresso, stirring it with the little spoon he handed her, while Mack drank his black.

She made a face. “I don’t know how you can drink that without a hint of sweetness in it.”

“I like the unadorned flavor of the coffee.”

“So do I. But I like mine sweet.”

He grinned, one brow up. “Some like it sweet. Some prefer it bold and steamy.”

Surely he hadn’t meant that to sound the way it had. As if he were talking about something that had nothing to do with coffee.

Trying to make herself think about something other than sex, she asked, “How long do you think the surgery will take?”

“It depends on whether those scissors have

done anything other than just create that chest wound. If he's having to cobble together blood vessels, it may take a little longer."

She nodded. "I was amazed at how well she held it together."

"She's a pretty tough lady. She grew up under difficult circumstances but was determined to live differently—to make a better life for her daughter."

"And she has. I hope I'm half the mother that she's been. I've only met Sally a time or two, but she seems to be following in her mother's footsteps."

His smile faded. "You're going to make an awesome mother, Lainey."

"How do you know?"

"It's in the way you talk about your pregnancy. In the way you didn't care what I thought when you were telling me that you were going to carry the pregnancy to term."

"Oh, I did care. But I had already made the decision and nothing you said would have changed my mind."

"Don't I know it. Been there. Tried that."

This time there was no doubt he was talking about something other than the subject at hand. He was talking about their breakup and her determination to move to Boston and take the new job. He hadn't told her *not* to take it, to be honest. He'd simply asked if she'd thought it through, and Lainey had immediately bristled. Would she have been so set on accepting the offer if his words hadn't set her off?

Maybe not. But it was the instinctive way she'd dealt with her dad's veiled attempts to manipulate her into doing what he wanted. She wished she were a little more like Mack in that one area. Unflappable and steady, thinking things through before he did them.

But sometimes, it felt like he did so much thinking that he never actually got there when it came to change. He weighed out each and every little facet ad infinitum, and it used to drive her crazy. And not in a good way. But as for her part in their split, she hadn't handled her side of things in a good and healthy way either.

She sighed and leaned forward. "I'm sorry I hurt you back then, Mack. It had nothing to do with you or our marriage. I just felt like I…"

"Wanted more than both of those things?"

"That's not fair." And there she went, bristling all over again. "I wanted to explore something new and challenging. To see what I'm capable of."

And yet that had not worked out either. But to Mack's credit, he actually changed the subject rather than risk escalating the situation. "Have you made an appointment yet at the birthing clinic?"

She was relieved to be moving on from the current topic. "I was just thinking about that this morning. No I haven't, but I need to."

"Would you mind if I come to it with you once you've done that? I know we haven't talked about it, but I'd like to hear what the doctor has to say about..." His words faded away.

"About my age? About any special considerations that come along with that?"

"If you must know, yes. I'd like to know what we're up against before it gets here."

Again, there was that need to examine things from every angle.

She thought for a minute. Did she really want that every time she went to one of her appointments? "Are you going to hover the entire pregnancy?"

"No." One side of his mouth went up in that irresistible way of his. The way that made her own mouth water. "I promise I'll only hover this first time."

She was skeptical and she was pretty sure her face showed it. "Somehow I don't believe you." She paused. "But it's nice to know you care."

"I do care. I want this baby to have the best chance possible."

So it was only because of the baby. Even

though that made sense—that all caring about Lainey's well-being had ended when their divorce was finalized—it still made her feel sad somehow, and she wasn't sure why. They were divorced; she'd lost any right to expect him to care about her as a person once those papers had been signed. And she'd certainly played a part in what had happened. A big one, she'd come to realize.

And even so, she gave voice to words that she probably should have left unsaid. "You can come. But please don't try to tell me what to do or how I should be doing it."

"I won't. Unless you try to guzzle down a box of wine."

The unexpectedness of his comment made her laugh. "Boxed wine? When have I ever sipped—not guzzled—alcohol that's packaged in cardboard? I'm much more a daiquiri girl, anyway."

"I remember. Everything."

His voice was low and gruff, and suddenly the atmosphere changed. Got heavier. And she knew why. How many times had he commented on how sexy it was to kiss her after she'd had a few sips of her favorite adult beverage? How often had she peered at him over the top of her glass as she tasted the sweetness of strawberries on her tongue and shared that taste with him later as she slid it between his lips and let him suck on it?

Oh God. Her eyes closed for a second, trying to banish the remembered sensations. She could almost feel…

"Lainey, don't."

She looked at him and saw the heat in his gaze. The knowledge that he knew what she was thinking about. What she wanted from him. "Lordy, I can't help it. I wish I could but…"

"I know. Hell, Lainey, I know." He leaned across the small table, his palm cupping the back of her head and staring into her eyes. "Because I'm on exactly the same page."

Then he did exactly what she'd dreamed of him doing ever since Boston. He kissed her.

Mack wasn't sure what prompted him to reach for her. Dammit! Yes he was. It was the way she'd responded to his comment, like she'd known exactly what he was referring to after her daiquiri comment. And she'd been right.

And despite the edge of the table that was now digging into his gut, the last thing he wanted to do was to pull back and leave the heaven of her mouth. And the taste of her coffee on her lips was making a believer out of him that sweeter was indeed better.

Lainey had always been a great kisser,

switching from receiving to giving at the slightest whim. It sometimes made him dizzy trying to keep up with her. This time was no different. She was no longer just letting him hold her in place, she was actively angling her mouth under his in a way that made his whole body tense in readiness, ever so hopeful that it knew where this was headed.

But it wasn't. Not here in a café where anyone could walk in at a moment's notice. But maybe they could…

As if his thoughts had made it happen, a sharp knock at the door had them both jerking back from the other. Lainey's eyes were glazed and the hair she'd held back with a clip was now flowing around her shoulders in sweet disarray. Bedroom hair. The kind that had often made him linger in bed for much longer than he should have.

The knock came again.

"Th-that might be Maria's daughter." Lainey's voice was soft, the whispered words difficult to make out. But he finally got what she was trying to say. Then she slid from her chair and scooped something up from the floor.

When she twisted her hair and resecured it, he realized it was her clip. It was as if in that single act, she reset the whole scene, transforming it from sexy oasis into what could have been a formal meeting.

Formal wasn't the kind of meeting he'd had in mind. And yet that in itself was ludicrous.

He stood as well and headed for the door, wondering what the hell he had been thinking. It was ridiculous to be making out with his ex-wife right after rendering aid to someone in distress. It seemed inappropriate.

Seemed? Hell, it *was* inappropriate no matter when or where it happened, and he'd better keep a better handle on that libido of his. Lainey was not only his ex, she was also pregnant with his child because of things exactly like today. And since neither one of them wanted to get back together, this kind of shit needed to stop right now.

He opened the door, and it was indeed Maria's daughter. He recognized her from her own shifts here at the café.

"Did the hospital get word to you? About your mom, I mean."

"Yes, I just went to check on her. She's still in surgery, and the nurse at the desk said they weren't expecting to be done for another half hour or so. You guys are the ones who helped her?" She peered past him and must have spotted Lainey.

He stood aside to let her in. "Yes, we gave

her first aid while waiting for the surgeon to get here."

"Thank you so much for that. I can't believe that happened. They said she fell on something. Was it a knife?"

Lainey offered her her chair. "Do you want something to drink? Coffee? Mack knows how to work the machine, if so."

"No. I'm fine."

He responded. "It was a pair of scissors, but we're hopeful that she'll be fine. We asked the surgeon to keep us in the loop."

"Scissors. God! I'll let you know as well. Mom would want me to keep the shop open, and that way I'll bc right here when she comes out of surgery. Is there anything I need to do as far as…um, cleaning up from her accident?"

"No, I think that was all taken care of," Lainey said.

She smiled. "By you two, I'm assuming?"

His ex-wife laid her hand on the woman's shoulder. "Hey, it was the least we could do. Your mom was more worried about the café than she was about herself."

"She's always been that way. She was like that with me and my brother as well. She always put us before everything else in her life. And now that she has a grandchild on the way…"

Mack realized he'd almost missed the meaning of her words. Maria's daughter was expecting. Now that she'd said it, he could see it. How long before Lainey's condition would be just as noticeable?

In fact, he'd pretty much forgotten she was pregnant when he'd kissed her. But sooner or later it would be impossible to miss.

"Congratulations," Lainey murmured. "Your mom must be thrilled."

"We both are. Not to mention my husband. If my mom's injury had been worse..."

It had been pretty bad, but Mack wasn't going to say that. If those scissors had gone in a little to the left, they could have hit her heart. Then this scene would have looked very different.

But it wasn't. And he needed to look at the positive side instead of focusing on the negative all the time.

Lainey hurried to reassure her. "The surgeon seemed optimistic. And even when we were trying to weigh our options as far as first aid goes, your mom was cracking jokes."

"That sounds just like my mom." Sally glanced at the door. "And now I'd better get this place opened back up before she gets out of surgery and kicks my butt for not working."

This time it was Mack who said, "Somehow I don't think she would."

"You're right. She wouldn't. But I don't want

to let her down. Thanks again for everything. And if you hear something before I do, would you please keep me updated?"

"Absolutely."

And with that, Lainey headed out the door, leaving Mack to take their paper coffee cups over to the trash before following her out. By the time he stepped through that door, she was long gone. And he should be glad. Because that meant he didn't have to issue an apology. At least not yet. But he made a mental note. No more leaning across tables to get closer to her and definitely no more kissing.

But as he'd seen firsthand, that was easier said than done. And now that he knew it wasn't only on his side, was it going to make things easier in that they were both aware of the dangers? Or would it make it that much harder to keep his hands—along with every other body part—to himself?

CHAPTER FIVE

IT HAD TAKEN Lainey a full week to get her first prenatal appointment at the new clinic. She'd debated on not telling Mack, but he had made it a point to tell her he'd like to be there, as long as she didn't object.

She didn't. But there was the matter of that kiss in the café that neither of them had brought up since it happened. And they'd worked together several times since then. But kind of like the problems in their marriage, it seemed easier just to ignore them than to tackle things head-on.

But Lainey didn't want to be the one to bring it up. And actually, she was just as happy that Mack hadn't said anything either. Obviously the chemistry was still there. Boy was it ever. Which struck her as kind of weird. Normally divorced couples couldn't stand being around each other, could they?

Not that she knew a whole lot of them. Lainey's had been the first divorce in their family. Or at least among her sisters, who were still with their partners. One of the couples wasn't married, but they were high school sweethearts who'd been together for close to twenty years. And her mom probably should have gotten a divorce but she'd stayed with him until he died.

She sat in the parking lot waiting for Mack. This was becoming a regular occurrence: her waiting on him. *Ugh!* Which brought up thoughts of Boston all over again and how she'd waited for something that never happened. She tried to shake free of that memory so she could focus on the here and now, like the fact that she'd gotten moved into her apartment, which had been exciting. Fortunately she'd been able to find one with two bedrooms, so it would do her for a good long while.

The birthing clinic looked very similar to its sister clinic. Not for the first time, she wondered who'd had the kind of money to bring these two centers into existence. Mack said it was an anonymous donor, and although there were some deep pockets in Austin, it seemed it would be harder to keep something like that a secret here than in, say, New York City.

Her doctor's name was Dr. Tracy Lindhart. She was an ob-gyn, and if Lainey were younger she might have felt more comfortable with a midwife, but she wanted to give the center as little cause to reject her as possible. Although why she was expecting them to do that, she had no idea. No one had called or questioned her age when she emailed her paperwork in.

She got out of her car and locked it and forced a smile as Mack did the same, although right now, she was kind of a nervous wreck. Not only about the appointment but about talking to her ex about things other than work. Because that's how they'd gotten through the last week…just keeping conversations limited to patients and treatments.

"How's it going?" she said.

"Pretty good. You?"

And that was that. In silence they headed toward the front door.

Maria had come through surgery just fine, and although she wasn't back at the café yet, her daughter said she should be back by next week. There'd been no complications from the scissors, which had been by no means sterile since she'd been using them to open up veggie packs. But at least it hadn't been raw meat or something worse. And Maria had told Sally how to make Lainey's favorite lavender-blend iced latte—the decaf version. Better yet, Sally had made one for herself and loved it so much that she promised it would be featured in their coffee-drink-of-the-week campaign. Mack wouldn't be able to pooh-pooh it then. Although she knew it was all in fun.

And until that kiss, they'd begun to joke around with each other again, something she'd sorely missed since moving up to Boston. No one there seemed to get her rather dark sense of humor, and one of her colleagues had actually looked at her in horror when she joked about having a porcelain doll in her house that her family swore was cursed. It wasn't, although they all remembered being creeped out by it as children when it sat on their grandmother's bed. These days, it sat in that same grandmother's antique rocking chair that had been handed down to Lainey almost ten years ago. Mack had made her put the doll in a guest room, saying he couldn't make love to her while it was in the room watching them.

But they'd laughed about it. He'd gotten her in a way no one else had. Not even her family. Maybe because her sisters and mom had always cringed when she went toe to toe against her father when he did something that she deemed unfair. And in the same way that Mack had understood her when she'd bristled at something her dad said, she'd understood his fraught relationship with Thom Morrison. At least she thought she had. Although she knew no one could truly understand except the person who'd lived through their difficult childhood.

Once inside the building, they went up to the reception desk. Of course, just like the people at the other clinic, these folks all knew Mack and greeted him as she gave one of them her name and signed in. She was pretty sure they were all wondering why Mack was accompanying her to the appointment. But for all they knew, she could be his sister. No. Not sister. It was probably pretty obvious that they weren't related by blood, although she knew that Mack really did have a half sister that she'd never met.

Then once they said her paperwork was all in order, she and Mack went and sat in a quiet corner of the waiting room. There were four other women there, some of whom were accompanied by someone and one who was here by herself, but her hand sported a wedding ring, so Lainey assumed she wasn't really doing this on her own.

According to Mack, she wasn't going to have to do this on her own either, although she was pretty sure she'd be the primary story reader at night. And if something happened in the middle of the night and Mack was on almost the other side of town from her apartment…

Wait. Did he still live in their house? She assumed he did, but maybe he hadn't been able to face it after the breakup.

"I never even asked. Are you still in the house?"

He blinked at her. "You mean the one we lived in?"

She nodded, a rock forming in the pit of her stomach.

"No. I sold it a year ago and bought something smaller."

That made her sad, although it shouldn't. She'd loved that house. Together they'd made so many improvements on it and made it their own. But had she really expected him to keep it? She probably wouldn't have if their positions had been reversed.

"That makes sense. I don't know why I asked."

"It's okay. It was just too big for one person."

They'd bought that house when they decided to try to have children. Three bedrooms, a large backyard and a year's worth of work and they'd declared it baby-ready. Only the baby was coming two years too late. If she'd gotten pregnant quickly would she have taken that job in Boston?

Probably not. But they'd tried for six months and nothing happened and both of them began to get irritable. And then that job offer had come. Maybe Lainey had looked at it as a way to escape the disappointment that came month after month. But she didn't think so. She'd truly been excited to have been approached by the team, who she found out later had been tipped off by one of her sisters who was a doctor at a different hospital in Austin. It had been in response to a flyer asking health care workers to name someone they considered the best of the best at their job. Hope had named Lainey.

"You're made for bigger things," Hope had told her. "You've never been happy just going with the status quo. Even Dad eventually saw that. He was proud of you," she'd shared at their father's funeral.

Lainey sighed. She hadn't actually talked to her sisters recently. She was sure they knew she was back in town thanks to her mom, but she knew her mother would not share the news of Lainey's pregnancy without her permission. She needed to tell them soon though. She'd been back for two weeks now. It was time. She just wanted to get through this appointment first and make sure things were going okay with the pregnancy.

"Alaina Thornton?" The door opened up, and she realized she was now the last person in the room, which seemed eerily quiet since neither she nor Mack had said much. She glanced at her watch. It was almost five o'clock, so that made sense. She was probably their last patient of the day.

"I'm here." She glanced at Mack, unsure if he planned on accompanying her into the back. But evidently he did, since he'd also climbed to his feet.

"Ready?" she whispered to him. He was probably as nervous as she was, if she had to guess. And she already missed the warmth of his leg that had been pressed close to hers as they sat side by side in the waiting room.

"Yep, let's go."

"Hi, Mack," the nurse said as they came through. The woman didn't ask how he was related to Lainey. She had to be dying to know though. But honestly, it wasn't Lainey's news to tell. Well, maybe it was, but she didn't want to announce him as the baby's father without talking to him about that first. She assumed he'd be all right with it, since he was here, but she didn't want to presume.

"Hello, yourself."

Lainey got on the scale, surprised that her weight hadn't changed more than it had, but then again, she'd been super busy between the move from Boston and work. But once they were in the room, Mack turned to her. "Shouldn't you have gained more by now? This is week ten, isn't it?"

"Not quite, but almost. I'm sure things are going to be popping out all over pretty soon." She didn't want to tell him that she'd lost close to fifteen pounds when she moved up north. It wasn't just because of missing her family and friends—and Mack. Everything was just different. The pace of life was much faster than it had been in Texas, and even the food had taken a bit to get used to. The regional differences had been surprising. And overwhelming. And between her Texas drawl and the accent of that area, even that had thrown her for a loop. But the folks at the hospital had been kind and had welcomed her in. For that she would always be grateful.

"Do you know the ob-gyn?" she asked.

"Which one do you have?"

He never asked her which route she'd decided to go. Maybe he thought it would be an invasion of privacy, but the lack of communication just served to remind her of how alone she might be in this process.

"Dr. Lindhart."

Just then the doctor herself came into the room. Young looking and with long red hair that was pulled into a high ponytail, she looked like she was fresh out of medical school, although she had to be at least thirty. But it still served to show that Lainey was not going to be a young mon this point in her life. Tracy sported wha like a wedding ring on her left hand, but her if she had chil- dren didn't seem appro

"Hi," she said. "You m Alaina." Her gaze swept to Mack. "And y "

"Mack Morrison. I'm the ba s father."

"Mack Morrison…" Her head ed. "That name sounds familiar."

Oh no. Mack hated it when people sked if he was related to Thom Morrison, but efore he could say anything the doctor snapped her fingers. "You work at Austin Memorial, don't you? ER?"

"Yep, that's me."

She had to admit, Mack looked relieved.

"You treated my sister a year ago. She fell off her bike after going too fast down a hill and broke her leg, not that I expect you to remember her."

The woman actually giggled, which did not seem in keeping with the sophisticated facade she presented. Lainey suddenly knew she was going to like this woman. She relaxed into her seat, realizing she'd been sitting ramrod straight to the point that her back was starting to hurt.

"I think I do remember her. She hit a fire hydrant and went over the handlebars? Compound fracture of the femur?"

“That’s my sist never does anything in half measures still riding bikes?”

He smiled. “ ll mad about the placement

“Yep, but sh nd now she swears that her of that hydr gerous than the performance bike is more d ained and shows.” horse that sh

“I don’t now if I exactly agree with that.”

“Me er. She says her horse would have jumpe that hydrant and continued on his way” Her look encompassed Lainey. “Anyway, I guess we should get on with why you’re here. Please call me Tracy, by the way. From what I understand you’re a doctor as well?”

“Yes. I just moved back to Austin from Boston. I work with Mack at the hospital’s main campus.”

“Great.” She consulted her tablet then frowned. “This says you’re at almost ten weeks? Any reason why you’ve delayed getting checked?”

Lainey was sure her age was going to come up at any second. “I should have, I know. But I was pretty busy getting ready to move across the country.” She decided to take the bull by the horns. “I’ll be thirty-nine when the baby is born, so I know that may come into play when it comes to deciding if I have the baby here at the clinic.”

…ing of going…

"I just thought that maybe the clinic would have stringent rules and…" She couldn't think of anything else so she let her voice fade away.

"We have a lot of women who are starting their families a little later. We can give you the same care as Austin Memorial provides. You've read our brochure."

Lainey nodded. "I have. And I have to admit, I'm kind of surprised. Will I be limited as far as my preference of birth experience?"

"Not that I can think of, unless there's a serious problem with the baby or if there are multiple fetuses or twin to twin transfusion syndrome or so forth. But those are things we can talk about a little further down the line. But today we need to get a baseline. That will include a sonogram, if you're okay with that."

Lainey hadn't even thought about the need for an ultrasound. She felt good other than an occasional queasy sensation in the morning. But it was never anything debilitating.

"Yes, I'm fine with it."

The thought of seeing their baby on a screen suddenly made this pregnancy seem much more real than it had over the past several weeks.

"Okay, I'm going to have you get undressed

and we'll do a full exam. Do you want Mack in here for that?"

The man had seen her naked for many years; it shouldn't have been an issue, but suddenly it was. Maybe because she was feeling much more vulnerable because of her condition. Or maybe that kiss in the hospital café was making her feel that way. But she'd told him he could be a part of all of this, so she'd better get used to it. "Yes, I'm okay with it as long as he is."

Why was she avoiding speaking directly to him? Because right now, having someone as a buffer seemed to be so much easier.

"I'm fine with it too."

But when she looked into his face, she thought she caught a tinge of red as if he too were slightly uncomfortable. Maybe they could talk about it when the doctor left the room so she could change.

That happened a moment later when Tracy stepped through the door to give her some privacy.

"Are you sure you want to stay?"

"I am."

Still, there was a curtain that she could draw in a small circle around herself, which she did. She quickly stripped off her clothing and put on the gown, keeping the opening in the front. Then she came out and sat on the exam table, putting the drape over her lap. Mack was studiously avoiding looking at her, which said he felt just as uncomfortable as she did. Someone tapped on the door. “Come in.”

That was faster than she expected, but maybe the ob-gyn just had the timing down to a science.

She lay back on the table when directed, and once a nurse joined her in the room, the doctor did an internal exam. Fortunately, with the way the table was situated, Mack couldn’t really see anything. An unexpected blessing, but one that she wasn’t going to question.

A minute later the doctor withdrew her instruments and nodded. “You’re definitely pregnant, although I’m sure you never doubted that. But you’d be surprised at how the body can play tricks.”

Yes it did. Like in the bar, when it said she needed something that only Mack could give. And boy had he ever. Or when she’d admitted to the attraction in the café. This thing between them, even if it was only skin-deep, was becoming harder and harder to ignore. At least for her.

The nurse cleaned up the area and got the sonogram machine ready, lubricating both Lainey’s stomach and the wand.

"Depending on what I see here, we may opt to do an internal ultrasound as well."

Something else Lainey hadn't thought of. Maybe she'd been in some kind of denial or something.

She took a measurement and wrote it down. "How much did you weigh on average before you got pregnant? Just so we can chart it."

If she told the truth and gave her weight before she moved to Boston, it would look suspicious, like it had to Mack when she'd stepped on that scale. "I had actually lost a bit of weight right before I got pregnant." She named the number, and when she chanced a glance at Mack, there was a frown. Whether it was worry or simply filing the information in his brain, she had no idea. He hadn't noticed the loss in the hotel room that night, but then again they'd both had a little more to drink than they probably should have.

Tracy nodded. "Okay, so you've gained about what I would have expected you to. So let's get a look at that little one."

Punching in Lainey's and Mack's names and dates into the machine, she then sat on a stool and wheeled it over to the exam table, where she pressed it to Lainey's belly and began dragging it through the lubricant in search of their baby. A rhythmic swishing noise came through just as a clear bubble emerged from the dark screen. Lainey could just make out a tiny form inside the bubble.

"There you are," Tracy said. "Good strong heartbeat too."

Lainey stared at the screen, whispering, "It's hard to believe this is real."

A sudden movement from the side caught her attention, and when she glanced at Mack, he had his phone out. "Sorry. I have to take this." He got out of his chair and left the room.

Had she missed the sound of his phone ringing? Maybe he'd had it on vibrate. But there was something about how fast he got out of there that made her think it didn't have anything to do with the call and more to do with her pregnancy.

She looked at Tracy, but she hadn't seemed to notice, commenting that she only saw one fetus and that from where she sat, everything looked good.

Trying to force herself to turn her attention back to the screen, she tried her best not to worry about what Mack was thinking. Or what he might be doing.

He'd had to get out of there. As soon as the sound of the baby's heartbeat filled the room, his own had tripped over itself as a sudden sense of panic burst through him. He was in a clinic seeing the physical evidence that he was going to be a father. Coming so quickly after that kiss in the café, the whole situation had overwhelmed his system. Guilt. Happiness. Confusion. And regret.

It was the last one that really got to him. Some of his actions hadn't exactly been commendable when she'd been asked to take on that job in Boston.

He hadn't been the most supportive husband on the planet. And now he had to decide what kind of father he was going to be. Except he wasn't sure. What if he screwed it up like his and Lainey's dads had done? What if he couldn't handle the simplest task—like changing diapers or rocking the baby to sleep?

Would Lainey even let him do those things? They hadn't really discussed who would do what. Would he keep the baby overnight? No. Probably not if Lainey was going to nurse, and when they'd decided to try for a baby of their own, she indicated that she would.

They could always share a household for a while so he could help her through those early days.

No. He doubted she'd want that either. And since they couldn't seem to keep their hands off each other, that probably wasn't the best idea. She'd probably want her mom to stay with her, anyway. Which meant he would be missing out on so much. So very much.

He slouched in a chair in the waiting room, pretty disgusted with himself. There'd been no urgent phone call. He'd lied. Already. And the baby wasn't even born yet. How was that for giving Lainey the support she needed? He should go back in there.

No. But he would stay here and confess the truth when she came out. Mack was a person who needed to know his role. In both his job and his personal life. He'd thought he knew both until Lainey had wanted to move to Boston. Then he'd felt like he was free-falling and that everything he thought he knew was dissolving right in front of his eyes. It hadn't been. At first. But then his own inability to bend and change had brought the universe down on himself and his marriage along with it.

He wouldn't blame Lainey if she said, "Forget this!" and stormed out of the doctor's office. But he hoped she wouldn't do that. He hoped she'd stick around and let him try to explain.

Five minutes later she came out of the door. Her eyes scanned the space and saw him immediately. She came over and sat next to him in the waiting room. "Are you okay?"

"Not really. There was no phone call."

"I know."

"I panicked."

She smiled and touched his hand. "I know that too. I felt a little panicky myself, but it would have been a little more awkward for me to leave the room."

That brought a smile out of him, even though the situation was not at all funny. But he decided to tell her the truth. "Can we sit down sometime and spell out my role in the baby's… Wait, there's not more than one, is there? I kind of left before that had been established."

"There's only one baby." She eyed him and her easy smile had faded. "I'm not sure I understand what you mean about spelling out your role. Do we need to do that?"

"I don't want to be left out, Lainey. I saw that baby appear and thought of all the things I wasn't going to be able to do. Like rock him or her to sleep at night. Like give baths or kisses good-night."

Her eyes cleared. "I get it. When you left the room, I thought maybe you'd changed your mind about being involved."

"No. I want it even more now."

"Me too." She looped her arm through his

and squeezed before letting go. "I'll do my best not to leave you out. But I think the office is closing and any further discussion needs to happen somewhere else. And I think I know where."

They drove to Lainey's new apartment, and she motioned him to pull in beside her. Rolling down her window, she said, "Two-bedroom apartments have two parking spaces. It works out well, don't you think?"

She wanted to show him the place and let him see where the nursery was going to go. He was a little surprised she wasn't going to look for a house of her own rather than continue renting, but that was her decision, not his. And the complex was nice enough. It had a pool that he could see through one of the corridors off the parking lot. Hopefully there were safeguards in place. Then he shook his head. It didn't matter. It was doubtful that she'd find herself here in three or four years. She'd either have another place, or she'd be remarried, a thought that made him uneasy. A man who actually lived with her would automatically be the baby's father figure, wouldn't he?

She said she wouldn't leave him out and he believed her. Or at least he believed that her intentions were to keep him involved. Who knew exactly what would happen two or three years down the road?

They walked to a flight of stairs and he frowned. "There's no elevator?"

"Yes, but I'm not afraid of a flight of stairs. Are you?"

"Of course not. I was just wondering how you were going to manage hauling a stroller up the stairs if there wasn't one."

"There is. Come on."

They went up the stairs and came out on a landing. "Right or left?"

"I'm five doors down to the right."

He was a little uneasy about the apartment complex having doors on the exterior of the building rather than all residents going through the interior to get to their places. It seemed a little less secure. But this was what Lainey wanted, and he really didn't have a choice in it. Maybe he should have kept the house, then he could have asked her to stay with him until the baby was a year or two old. It had been large enough that they could have pretty much had their own wing, with the primary bedroom on one side of the house and the others on the other side. But to ask her to move in with him now—in his new place—would be uncomfortable for both of them. It had two bedrooms, but one was tiny and set up as an office.

And he didn't think she would agree no matter what. So he wasn't going to ask. They would figure it out.

"And here it is." She pulled out her key and opened the front door. The corridor looked out over the pool and courtyard, and there looked to be an area for entertaining family and friends. "You'll have to forgive the boxes. I haven't finished unpacking yet."

That was surprising, but then again, she'd been pretty busy since arriving back in Austin. But when he walked in, there wasn't a box in sight. "I thought you said there were boxes."

"There are, believe me. They're all in what will be the nursery. Let's head that way."

The apartment was cool and certainly seemed to be well maintained. He followed her down the hallway into the second bedroom. All that was in there right now was an antique rocking chair with… He couldn't hold back a laugh. "Are you sure you want her in the baby's room?"

Lainey smiled back at him, and her glance went to the doll sitting in her grandmother's rocker. "You'd better be careful insulting her. She might just follow you home."

"And that sounds like the scene from a

movie. No thanks. I think she and I have made our peace."

She looked at him and paused. "And how about you and me? Have we made our peace?"

CHAPTER SIX

LAINEY WAITED FOR his response, afraid to breathe. She hadn't meant to ask the question; it had just popped out. But she found she very much wanted to know the answer to that question.

"I'm hoping we can. Maybe the baby can help us with that." He didn't quite meet her eyes.

She hadn't expected him to propose or say that he still loved her, and she didn't want that. But she missed his friendship and the easy companionship they'd once had. She probably shouldn't expect that to come back—after all, she knew she'd hurt him back then. But she couldn't allow anyone to shame her into doing what they wanted.

And he hadn't. She could see that now. To even think otherwise was doing Mack a huge disservice. He was nothing like her dad. He was nothing like his dad either. So why was her knee-jerk reaction to act as if he were? Hadn't she been the one to dictate to him what he should do when she expected him to move to Boston just like that?

But if she'd hurt him by leaving, he'd hurt her by not even coming to visit her even one time after she moved. By not suggesting they meet somewhere halfway to discuss things. But then she'd done neither of those things either. She hadn't come home to Austin for Christmas that year.

He'd wandered over to look at some boxes of furniture she'd bought from one of the big Swedish retailers in the area. "Need any help putting some of this together?"

And maybe this could be their way toward peace. If she included him as much as possible in the things related to the baby. "I would love some. I looked at the instructions for the crib, and it has a crazy number of pieces. I was too afraid to look at the rest of what I bought."

"Do you have some tools?"

"You mean, like, do it now?"

"I have the time, if you do. If not, I can come back."

She thought through what she had in her pantry as far as food went. She could make some Alfredo, which he'd always loved. "I'll tell you what. If you're sure you want to tackle one of those boxes, I can make us some dinner."

"That sounds like a good trade-off. With one caveat."

She tensed, expecting him to say that he didn't want anything she might fix. "Okay, what?"

"That you check on me every half hour or so to make sure she—" he pointed at the rocking chair "—doesn't try to pull any funny business."

And just like that, everything was okay. Like the light at the end of a very dark tunnel.

It was so nice to have someone to joke with about things again. She patted the doll on the head. "She's been a good girl for quite a long time. As long as you're nice to her, you should be good."

"And if I'm not?"

"Then you might not want to turn your back on her." With that, she scooted out of the room, her sense of relief the biggest she'd felt in quite a while. And she could only hope her luck continued. Because the way he'd smiled at her had made a warmth bloom inside of her that continued to glow as she gathered stuff to make the Alfredo she'd promised him.

Fifteen minutes later, she heard an oath and a large crash. Dropping her whisk, she hurried to the bedroom to find Mack on the floor nursing his thumb. There was blood on one of the rungs of the crib. "What did you do?"

The way he looked at her made her realize how that sounded. "I meant to yourself. Not to the furniture. You're bleeding."

"It's nothing. The screwdriver slipped, and I ripped part of my nail off."

"Let me see." Moving closer, she took his hand and held it in hers, turning it over so she could see. True to his word, part of his thumbnail had ripped far enough down to have disturbed some tiny blood vessels, which were still oozing. "Come with me."

"I'm fine. I'll just wash my hands and—"

"Yes, *we'll* wash your thumb and then I'll bandage it."

They got to the bathroom, and Lainey turned on a tap, mixing cold and hot water until the stream was lukewarm. "Here, stick it under there, while I get some ointment and a Band-Aid."

He did as she asked, holding his thumb under the water. "Dammit."

"What?"

"Nothing. It just stings."

She smiled again. For such a big stoic guy, he'd never had the highest pain tolerance. And it actually helped her to see him as human rather than some superhero or robot who felt nothing.

She came back with some antibiotic ointment. The kind that had a touch of lidocaine in it to help with the pain. She also had a pair of nail clippers. "I'm going to need to cut a little of that back so it doesn't rip any more than it already has."

"If you just slap a Band-Aid over it, it should be fine."

"Don't be silly."

They stood there for a few seconds staring at each other before he grinned. "Okay, go ahead. Are you sure you're not taking after Annabelle in there?"

It was Mack's pet name for her doll, the idea coming from a horror movie that had a doll with that name.

"Only in the best possible way." She held out her hand for his thumb.

With a sigh, he laid his hand in hers and she put the ointment on first, figuring the lidocaine in it couldn't hurt anything and maybe it would dull the pain he'd feel from her pulling on his nail.

She slid her clippers beneath the ragged part, knowing that she couldn't cut it all the way across because that would hurt like the devil. Instead she just clipped a very narrow slice straight up the nail. Glancing at his face, she asked if he was okay.

"Just finish it." She tried not to laugh at the tight pained sound to his voice. He hated to look weak, she knew from experience, but he hated being in pain even more.

She kept going, and when she reached the top, she rounded the corner just like she would have with anyone who came to the ER with this particular injury. Not that many did.

"Oops, I'll be right back." She forgot that she'd been whisking the sauce in the kitchen when he'd called out. By the time she got there, it was bubbling, but not ruined. She whisked it and turned the burner down to low.

She got back to find that Mack had gotten the bandage undone and was winding it around his thumb. Her brows went up. "Good thing I was done with that."

He grinned at her. "Oh, you were 'done,' even if you weren't done."

"Chicken."

"I will admit to that."

Lainey shook her head. "And you're an ER doc?"

"I'm not a chicken about other people's wounds. Just my own."

"Well, don't worry about the furniture. We have about ten minutes until dinner's done."

"Oh no. I am going to finish that crib. Even if I have to enlist Annabelle's help."

"You won't have to. Are you okay with eating on the floor of the nursery? I can help you and we can eat in between swear words."

"I never got the appeal of this company."

"Their stuff looks great. It's got clean lines, and most pieces are white so they appeal to the masses—as in me. You'll see, once we get it together."

She and Mack headed their separate ways, and once she had dinner ready, she put heaping portions into two bowls and sprinkled them with Parmesan cheese. Then she went back to the nursery and handed him both of the plates. "Don't let Annabelle eat mine. I'm going to get a couple of glasses of sweet tea."

She didn't ask if he wanted one, because she knew it was the one drink that he didn't mind sugar in. He liked it as sweet as she did, in fact. Stopping to stuff her hair back into her clip, she picked up the glasses and carried them back to the bedroom. Then they sat to eat.

Mack nodded his approval as he twirled his fettuccine, pausing to stab a piece of spinach before he put it in his mouth and chewed. "I haven't had this in ages."

"I hope it's as good as you used to say it was."

"Better. What's the saying? Absence makes the heart grow fonder."

Except when it came to her, it seemed. Because her absence in his life while she'd been in Boston hadn't elicited any kind of reaction in him. Not good. Not bad. Just a silence that had spoken louder than anything he might have said. She'd gotten the message loud and clear. And when she could stand it no longer, she filed for divorce.

She'd halfway thought maybe she'd be able to find love again in Boston, but instead she found herself overwhelmed by a sense of apathy. She just wasn't interested. Not in men. Not in food. And not in her job after the initial discovery period was over. She just hadn't cared.

And now that she was back in Austin?

Well, if her doctor was worried about weight, she needn't have been. Lainey found that her appetite was back. She was a voracious eater, actually. And she loved her job again. And she…

She stopped that thought right in its tracks. She wasn't interested in Mack again. Because down that road lay a whole lot of heartache.

Mack's plate was empty. He hadn't lied when he said he'd missed this. "More?"

"Yes, please. I'll put a couple more of these rungs on while you're getting it."

She set down her plate and went and dished him up another helping, glad that she'd decided to cook the whole box of pasta.

Taking it back to the room, she surveyed the scene as she handed him his food and sat back down. "This reminds me of when we were moving into our house and we were trying to unpack and eat and get things put away all at the same time. We ended up laughing and unable to get much done." She looked at him. "But we had fun, didn't we?"

"We did."

Things got awkward again, maybe because the memories she'd dredged up for both of them were bittersweet. There'd been a whole lot of good mixed with things that were downright painful.

Mack took a few bites and then put his plate down and went back to work. He had one side of the crib done. "Only five hundred and sixty pieces left to go."

"You eat and I'll take over for a few minutes."

It was less than a few minutes before she was as frustrated as Mack had been. Probably more because she had a lot less patience than her ex did. "Well, damn. This is terrible."

He looked at her as he shoveled another bite in his mouth, waiting until he had swallowed before responding. "I know. Are you going to furnish this whole room with more of these?"

"Well, I had my eye on a couple more items, but not anymore. I'd rather build the shelving unit from scratch than you having to go through this again…once all of this furniture is put together."

That did get him to laugh. "Thanks for having pity on me. Does that mean I'm being drafted?"

"If I had to put all of this together, the baby would end up sleeping on the floor."

"I'll make you a deal. You read the instructions and I'll do the grunt work."

Her nose crinkled. "Only if you promise to do the bare minimum of grunting."

"It's a deal. As long as you don't outlaw swearing."

She bumped her shoulder against his. "You'd better get all of that out before the baby is born. Because if I have to do without alcohol and caffeine during my pregnancy, you'd better get the cussing out of your system now."

"No more furniture from this place then, or I'm not making any promises."

Once they finished eating, she took their plates into the kitchen and dumped them into the sink and then went back to help him, the doll seeming to give her the side-eye as she walked by. Maybe she shouldn't stay in here once the baby was born. The last thing she needed was to have to take her child to therapy because of his or her mom's doll. But she could hope that they shared a sense of humor.

"Ready?"

"I am."

She picked up the set of instructions and tried to find where they were in the crib building process. "Okay, it looks like you're ready for the top side rail." She read what he was supposed to do, and he got that piece locked into place.

Once they started working together, things seemed to go better. Maybe the manufacturer should put a disclaimer on it saying that construction is much less painful when two people are tackling it together.

Maybe like life?

Except when two heads weren't better than one. When two people wanted two different things, life wasn't better. It became downright unbearable.

She tried to ignore that and just kept reading off the instructions to Mack when he was ready, his hands sliding over the pieces in a slow rhythm that was hypnotizing. And the concentration on his face was endearing, the tip of his tongue emerging from the corner of his mouth as he struggled with one of the harder pieces. It suddenly became hard for her to breathe. Fortunately, she had to inhale in order to read what came next. Then she paused and watched as he carried out her instructions.

In less than a half hour they had a crib.

Lainey helped him carry it to the wall under the window, and they set it into place and put the mattress inside. She stood back and looked at it. "Oh, Mack…"

"Yeah. I know. It makes it seem much more real, doesn't it?" He propped his fingers low on his hips—unaware of how sexy that move was—as he turned toward the boxes and perused what was left. "Well, now I'm riding high on the thrill of victory, let's tackle another one."

The next thing was the dresser. It also went better with both of them working together. They put that on the wall adjacent to the crib.

"The only other thing I have is the changing table, but that can wait for another day if you're tired."

"Nope. Let's get it out of the way." He glanced at his watch.

"Are you sure?" Was he itching to get out of here? Because if she had her way… Oh no. She was not going to visit that little corner of her mind. It was a place that always got her in trouble.

"I'd rather do it now, than walk away and let

the hard parts discourage me from something that could be rewarding if tackled in a timely manner."

Why did it sound like there was a life lesson in there?

But rather than try to dissect it, she just waited for Mack to tear open the last furniture box and dump the pieces out onto the floor. He handed her the instructions. "Well, at least we haven't had any leftover pieces."

"Look at you there, thinking on the positive side."

He smiled. "I *can* step out of my comfort zone from time to time."

At least they both knew their weak areas. Whether either of them was willing to work on them was another matter. But they were going to have to tackle some of those if they had any hopes of co-parenting this baby.

"Ready?" she asked.

"As I'll ever be. Let's time it and see how fast we can get it done."

For some reason that made her laugh. And she had trouble slowing down the mirth once it started. She finally got out, "That's what *she* said."

It was one of the key lines to a sitcom they'd watched together. It had been just as funny the second time around. And she and Mack had thrown that phrase at each other any time one of them said something that could be taken more than one way.

Mack shook his head. "Touché. But I don't think we were ever fast at that. Either one of us. We both liked to take our time. Make it last."

Oh, they were now treading on dangerous ground. She probably shouldn't have said what she did, but trying to explain it without using the actual phrase was almost impossible. And it had seemed funny. Until now.

"Yes we did."

They stared at each other for a few seconds before he broke eye contact first. "Let's not go there. So what's next?"

They got busy with the instructions, neither one of them saying anything for a while, and she mourned that rapport that had seemed—at least for a few minutes—almost normal. Until the conversation veered into subjects that should have been taboo. At least for them.

The truth was, they were both touchier than they had been about things. Things that didn't used to, now scraped across a nerve that was still raw from what had happened between them. And not just that time in the hotel room. It was from their breakup.

That specter would probably hang over them for the rest of their lives. Or at least until their child grew up and they didn't have to interact with each other as often. But that was eighteen long years away. And to wish away those years was to wish away a big part of her life. Of her child's life.

"Lainey? I'm waiting."

His words propelled her away from her thoughts and brought her back to the reality of what they were doing. "Put the drawer runner on the bottom of the first drawer."

"Really? They couldn't even do that for us?"

At first she thought he was actually mad, but then he waggled his brows at her and all was well with the world. Because she recognized that expression. It was one of exasperation, but there was also a hint of relief that she was there sharing in his pain.

"I guess not, or we would have been able to skip three pages ahead." She rifled the sheaf of paper. "And as it is, we still have plenty of steps to get through. I'm sure the tracks for the runners are next on our agenda."

"Perfect. Okay. I'm pretty sure I can handle the three other drawers, as long as the instructions have all the drawers alike."

She looked down. "Appears that way. Go, bab… Mack, go."

Oh Lord, she'd almost called him baby, the way she used to. How easy it was to sink into old familiar habits. But she'd better try to stay on her toes, or she would probably be sorry she didn't.

Her phone pinged. She retrieved it from the floor and glanced down at it. It was a phone number with a text from someone at the hospital.

Hi, Alaina, this is Daphne, one of the ER nurses. Is there any way you could come in today? We've had two doctors call off, and I don't want to bother Mack with it if I can find someone.

It was unusual for a nurse to do doctor staffing, so that either meant that whoever else was there was so busy that they couldn't stop what they were doing, or there wasn't a doctor there at all.

Of course. It'll take me a few minutes to change, then I'll be right there.

You're a lifesaver. See you soon.

When she put the phone down, she saw that Mack was looking at her. She wasn't sure how much to say, since Daphne didn't know he was with her. But he would wonder why she was going to leave in such a hurry. "I have to go to the hospital. You don't have to keep doing this, if you don't want to. I can put it together another time. You've done the hardest parts."

He looked at all the stuff lying on the floor with raised brows. "I doubt it. What's going on at the hospital?"

"Um…they're short-staffed and wanted to know if I could come in."

He grabbed his phone and looked at it. "I don't see anything on mine."

"She said she didn't want to bother you if she didn't have to."

His jaw tightened. "Who's she?"

She knew that look. Mack was nothing if not fair. But he also liked to go by the book, and Lainey was pretty sure that the protocol would have been to get in contact with Mack with problems like that. She wasn't sure why Daphne hadn't, actually. Except she remembered that Mack always put in more than his share of hours, and the nurse probably was doing what she said she was doing: trying not to bother him on his day off.

"Mack, don't get your panties in a wad. You know good and well that you do most of your paperwork after hours. The staff all knew it then, and they know it now. She is trying to be nice."

"For one thing, I don't wear panties. And for another, it doesn't matter. She should have contacted me. Okay. Don't tell me. But if they're that short-staffed then I'm going in with you."

Her brows raised. "And how are you going to explain how you suddenly knew about this?"

"I'll go in as if I'm there to do paperwork and I'll ask how it's going. Someone will undoubtedly tell me the truth."

Great. She should have just told him it was a problem with her mom or something. But then if he really did go to the hospital and saw her there, he'd know she lied. And one thing she'd always tried to do was tell him the truth. Even when it hurt like the devil.

He stood and dusted himself off. "Okay if I leave this here and we can take up where we left off later?"

She nodded, although something in her heart cramped. If only that applied in areas other than furniture building. She wasn't sure anyone could really start all over again though. Not after what had happened between them. "You go on ahead and I'll follow you in around fifteen minutes."

"If they're just one doctor short, I can cover it. I'll let you know if they truly need you. Was it Daphne?"

She blinked. How in the world had he guessed that?

"Never mind," he said. "I can see it in your

face. She's always been like a mother hen, clucking over everyone."

"Just let me go in, Mack. If it truly can be handled with just one extra doctor then one of us can leave. But if I don't show, she'll wonder why, and I would rather people not know we were together."

"They're eventually going to realize that you're pregnant and that I'm the father."

"Yes. They are. But I want to let those explanations happen on my terms and I want us to have decided on a story."

He frowned. "But it's not a story. This is real life."

"I know that, Mack." A wave of frustration built in her chest, removing the last couple of lighthearted hours. "Just go. I'll see you there, soon."

"Okay." He pocketed his phone and felt for his car keys before heading for the front door, leaving her standing in a room full of debris and unassembled parts and thinking about how much it looked like her life right now. She was a mess. A mismatched bunch of half-finished work with an instruction book that didn't do much good. And Mack's comments on those drawer runners was also true.

She glanced up. "Couldn't you have even put some of the little stuff back together for me?"

There was no answer. Which was kind of par for the course.

She guessed it was all up to her. Including getting dressed and heading out to the hospital, where she could hopefully help at least one person put their life back together. At least on a physical level.

CHAPTER SEVEN

IT WAS A good thing Mack had come. Daphne had met him at the desk and confessed that she called Lainey in. She hadn't wanted to bother him because he took so few days off.

His irritation evaporated. The crew in the ER really did take care of each other. Daphne went on. "Jack happened to come by, and we grabbed her to help. Just an FYI, Dr. Lacy kind of stormed out of here after having a difficult patient and said she was done. I think she was serious. If so, any chance we can ask Jack to join the department on a full-time basis?"

Jaqueline—Jack—Elliot was one of the Austin M's in-house doctors who worked the ER when they were truly shorthanded. She was ideal with children and gifted in the area of pediatric trauma medicine. They'd called her to handle several of those cases, and she'd always instinctively known the best ways to treat them. She had briefly approached him last week asking if he would consider her for a permanent spot on the team once Carter Jones retired, but then Glenda had bypassed him—much the way Daphne had bypassed him today—and asked Lainey to step into his shoes instead. He'd been the one who had to tell Jack that the position had been filled already. But maybe now…

Or there was another option. Sofie from the emergency clinic had said they were starting to get swamped as well. So maybe they could put her there. But then again, they were trying to staff those positions with people who weren't already at Austin M.

He glanced at Daphne. "Don't ever be afraid to call me. I want to help when you're short." After all, he didn't have a social life to speak of anymore. When Lainey had left for Boston, the hospital had by necessity taken up that empty part of his life. And now it pretty much ruled his days. And he hadn't complained. He'd needed it. More than he would ever admit to anyone.

"Okay." The woman smiled at him, but he didn't believe her for a minute. Daphne had always had a mind of her own, but she was a damned good nurse and they needed her. And not just for her nursing skills, but also for her administrative prowess. Although he'd chafed at it today, he appreciated her initiative and willingness to find a way when it seemed there wasn't one.

He tried to cover his butt about having been with Lainey, since his ex probably wouldn't appreciate him saying anything. "Did Lainey say when she was going to be here?"

"She said to give her about fifteen minutes to change and then she'd be in. I wouldn't have asked except there was an accident involving a car and a bicyclist. Jack is still with that patient."

He nodded. "Okay, give me someone."

The patient he got was a man in his late forties who was holding a blood-soaked rag to his forehead.

"Ouch," Mack said. "Do I dare ask what's under that?"

"My wife hit me upside the head with a two by four."

Mack frowned, until the man said he was kidding. Not really, but he'd been kidding about the implied intent. "We were building a new closet in our bedroom and she was bringing me a piece of lumber. She tripped over our dog, just as I was coming to get the piece of wood, and it hit me in the head." He shrugged. "She feels terrible. I just wanted to tape it together with a Band-Aid, but she insisted we come in. She's in the waiting room. She can't stand the sight of blood. She almost fainted when my head started to bleed."

"Well, let's see what's under that."

Mack slipped on a pair of gloves and peeled away the blood-soaked cloth. "When was your last tetanus shot?"

The man grinned. "The last time I got hurt, which was probably six months ago. I shot a nail through my hand with a nail gun."

"Ah…okay." It wasn't up to him to tell the man he might want to rethink his hobbies. But at least he was up to date on his tetanus booster.

The gash was about four inches wide, and there was already some ugly bruising around it. "I hate to tell you, but this needs more than a Band-Aid. You're going to need a few stitches."

"Dammit. I hate it when the wife is right."

Mack tried not to think about the fact that over the last two years he'd wondered if Lainey had been right in expecting him to move and that he might have been wrong in dragging his feet. Yes, his dad had yanked his boys out of their schools on a moment's notice without giving a thought to how it might affect them. Mack could have understood if they were in dire straits and his father had to do it to keep the family going, but Thom Morrison had already been wildly wealthy by that time. He simply got bored and didn't care who had to pay the price when he decided a new locale was in order.

Not something he needed to think of right now.

Lainey stuck her head in the door. "Need any help?"

"I need to suture this. Is there a nurse available to set up, do you know?"

"They're all helping patients. But there's a little bit of a lull in the waiting room, so we should catch up pretty soon. I can get you set up."

He didn't argue, just worked on getting a syringe filled with a numbing agent so he could get the laceration cleaned out and ready for stitching. "This is going to sting."

The man hissed out a breath, but other than that he was quiet as Mack did several needle sticks around the outside of the wound. Then he worked on cleaning the blood away and irrigating the wound to make sure there was no debris in there that would impede healing. By that time, Lainey had a tray ready with the suture material and a sterile dressing to put on afterward.

"Can I get you to lie back on the table and turn your head toward me?"

The man did as he asked, and Mack sat on the stool and pulled the tray over with him. He checked that the lidocaine had taken effect before picking up the pre-threaded curved needle and taking the first stitch. Fortunately the cut wasn't in an area of high motion, like over a joint, so the sutures should hold, unless infection set in. Hopefully that wouldn't happen though.

Daphne poked her head in. "Need me for anything? I just finished with my patient."

Smiling at the woman, Lainey said, "Unless you need me out there right now, I can help with this one. I know you've been swamped."

"Thanks. I'll go check on Jack. They're waiting on an ortho and neuro consult, and she doesn't want to leave the patient until someone gets there. It looks like everyone is busy. There's a big Grand Prix race today, and the local hotels are full. And there was a full moon last night."

That explained some of the extra patients. Austin was a busy place anyway, but it also housed one of the biggest Formula 1 racing tracks in the country. He wondered if Rhett was there today. He hadn't heard from his brother since that cryptic phone call last week.

Not something he needed to think about right now. If his brother wanted to get in contact with him, he would.

Mack also didn't need to be thinking about

how he always seemed to expect the other person to contact him rather than the other way around. He hadn't tried getting in contact with Lainey after she'd left, giving himself the same argument: if she wanted to talk to him she'd call. Only she hadn't. And neither had Mack.

He placed the final suture and forced his mind to stay on his patient and off his problematic relationships.

"Okay, I think we've got you put back together. You can sit up, but take your time."

Their patient sat up, and Lainey came over to dress the wound and tape it. "You can probably take this off tonight to let the air get to it, but it looks good."

Was she surprised that Mack still knew how to suture a wound? He didn't do as much patient work as he used to because of his position, but he still tried to spend a large amount of time in the ER working with patients. It's why he went into emergency medicine in the first place.

He gave her a look, and she tilted her head as if she had no idea why. And maybe she didn't. She did say that her job had not been exactly what she'd hoped for and that the administrative side of it had not been her favorite thing in the world. It wasn't his either, but he knew it needed to get done, and he tried not to let that be the main part of his job. But maybe Lainey hadn't had a choice. Every hospital was different in how much latitude they allowed their doctors to have in making decisions. It could be the hospital in Boston micromanaged more than they did at Austin M. But with a hospital as huge as that one was, they probably did need to run a tighter ship since there were so many people and components to manage.

He finished up the chart and let his patient head on his way while he helped Lainey get the room cleaned up and ready for the next patient. There were people who did that, but when things were super busy, he tried to pitch in wherever he could, and he knew Lainey had been like that as well. One area in which they'd been super compatible.

But not the only area. As made obvious by her pregnancy. And by the sexy comments they'd tossed back and forth at her apartment. It had felt right in a way that it shouldn't. And yet he'd wanted it to continue. Wanted the words to morph into action. He blew out a breath. Not something he should be thinking about right now.

"If you're good," she said, "I'm going to see if there are more patients who need to be seen. Can I send whoever the doctor on duty is on a break?"

"I think Dr. Elliot has been the only one

working, and from what I understand she's still with her patient who's in critical condition."

"Race days always make for busy hospital days."

"Yes they do."

As the track physician, he imagined that Rhett's days were busier too. He couldn't even imagine some of the horrific injuries his brother had seen. But then again, it wasn't something that they'd talked about much. His brother had shifted from job to job over the years, but racing seemed to have stuck. And Mack wasn't sure if he was happy about that or not. Because it wasn't just the doctor part that Rhett was involved in. He also liked to race. Which was probably part of the reason they didn't have much contact with each other. Mack could never seem to get inside Rhett's thought processes. Then again, Mack hadn't understood his dad either. Or Lainey, for that matter, although in the early part of their marriage he thought he had her all figured out. Until Boston had come along and wrecked any illusion of that.

Lainey left the room with a quick goodbye, and Mack sat on his stool for a moment or two and wondered where the hell he'd gone wrong with all of the relationships in his life. Because his father, his brother and his wife made three. Wasn't there a saying about that? If one person calls you a jackass, take it with a grain of salt. If a second person calls you a jackass, look in a mirror. If a third person calls you one, then you'd better go out and buy yourself a saddle.

He might very well be at the saddle-buying stage.

A half hour later, Lainey was at the nurses' station finishing up some paperwork on a patient she'd just seen when she saw Mack come out of one of the exam rooms followed by a woman who looked vaguely familiar, but she couldn't place her. She wore a stethoscope around her neck, so she obviously worked here. With long curly brown hair and a curvy figure, the woman was gorgeous. And Mack definitely knew her since both their faces were serious and it looked like they'd been in deep conversation.

She tried not to put any words in their mouths, but it was hard not to wonder.

Which was stupid. Lainey had no hold over him. Well, none except for her pregnancy, and the last thing she wanted to do was keep him from having relationships outside of their very tenuous connection. Except they'd kissed not very long ago. Surely he wouldn't jump from that to…

Mack spotted her and waved her over.

Great. She may have wondered who the person was, but she didn't want to be told flat out that this was someone he was dating. She'd rather just not know. But to refuse to go over there would let Mack know that this bothered her. Hell, she was reluctant to admit that fact to herself much less let him take one look at her face and guess the truth.

With legs that felt like lead, she moved toward the pair, who were no longer talking, but standing next to each other on the far wall watching her move toward them.

Talk about feeling self-conscious…

She made it over to them, and Mack took the lead. "I'm not sure if you guys have been formally introduced. This is Dr. Jack Elliot. She's been helping out here in the ER on days like today. Jack, this is Lainey Thornton. She just rejoined the Austin M family."

No mention that she and Mack had had a much deeper relationship in the past. It was as if he were purposely leaving that out.

But hadn't she asked him to? Hadn't she said she wanted to tell people on her terms?

"Nice to meet you, Jack. Sorry you had crazy duty today."

"It's kept me busy, which is something I needed. Especially today." The woman smiled, but there was something in her glance that said something was bothering her. But neither Mack nor the other doctor acted like they were involved in a way other than professionally. She allowed her tense muscles to release their grip on her stomach.

"Speaking of which…" Mack looked at her. "I just got off the phone with Dr. Lacy. She turned in her notice. Effective immediately."

"Oh no! It's not like we have a plethora of other ER doctors. And once Dr. Jones officially retires, we'll be down another one."

"That's what Jack and I were talking about. I need to put out an official notice that we're looking, and I've asked Jack to put in an application for the job. It needs to be official, and hospital bylaws require us to put a notice out for a week that there's an opening in the department. If there are no other applicants in that week, and I deem that the one person who applied is a good fit, then I can hire that person."

Meaning Jack.

Lainey crunched up her nose and smiled again at the woman. "I'm surprised we didn't scare you away with how chaotic it's been today."

"I like the busy atmosphere. It keeps me on my toes. Besides, it gives me something to think about besides my…" Her voice trailed away.

Lainey didn't say it out loud, but she got

where Jack was coming from. The ER gave her something else to think about other than her personal life. Which quite frankly was a mess right now.

The birthing clinic had called a few minutes ago and wanted to see her at her earliest convenience. The receptionist wasn't able to tell her why other than the fact that the doctor had a few more questions for her that she hadn't asked during that first appointment. She hadn't decided yet if she was going to tell Mack or not. What if Dr. Lindhart had taken a second look at her sonogram and found a problem that she hadn't seen when Lainey had been there? She'd promised she would call them back. After deciding what she was going to do about Mack.

"Hey, I get it," she said in response to Jack's comment. "There are days when I'd rather be anywhere but home."

"Exactly."

Mack glanced at her with a frown, but he didn't say anything. Instead he addressed Jack. "So I'll get that notice out there, but if you would, go ahead and turn in an application like we discussed. And I'll arrange for there to be an interview, depending on how many other applicants we have. I don't expect we'll have a whole rush of them. Emergency departments everywhere are going through a crisis right now. Doctors are looking to specialize in areas other than emergency medicine. But a lot of times, we are the first doctor some of our patients have seen in a long time. It's up to us to stand in the gap between family medicine and those other specialties."

Lainey nodded. "I can't count how many times a patient has come in for one thing only for tests to come back showing that the root cause is something else entirely. Like coming in for what was thought to be bronchitis only to find out the patient has stage four lung cancer. Those are the patients who are hard."

"I've had that happen before as well," Jack said. "And it's pretty awful to have to tell a parent who comes that the ache in their baby's arms is not growing pains, but is actually a neurodegenerative condition. I happen to love emergency medicine—except on those days." She glanced at Mack. "I'll get that application in today."

"Perfect. Thanks. I look forward to working with you."

Once the other doctor walked away, Lainey bit her lip. "You almost made it sound like a done deal."

"I pretty much expect it to be. But we'll wait and see what happens over the course of the next week."

She decided she needed to tell him. “Mack, the clinic called and they want to see me. They wouldn’t tell me why and…” She swallowed. “Well, I’m scared. What if they found something wrong with the baby?”

“I’ll go with you.” He didn’t wait for her to ask, he simply made it sound as if there were no question as to what he would do. And she appreciated it. It made her feel not so alone, although she needed to be careful not to lean on him too much. She’d done that once before and it had done her no good. In fact, it had hurt more than she’d wanted to admit that he hadn’t actually wanted to be there for her. At least not when it came to her move. And looking back, she’d been wrong—so very wrong—to have just up and assumed that he would be anxious to go with her. And now she saw why. Mack’s job fit him like a glove. If he were to leave, she was pretty sure the whole department would be devastated. And if not handled carefully, it could flounder without his leadership and spiral downward, its gold star rating vanishing in an instant.

“Thank you.”

He put his arm around her, taking it off again when Daphne rounded the corner and saw them, a slight smile curving her lips.

She wanted to warn the woman not to get her

hopes up, because Lainey wasn't. Mack was not interested in getting back together with her. He was simply trying to comfort her. But that he was quick to let her go after being caught said a lot. He didn't want people to assume they were back together.

She didn't want them assuming that either, did she? The fact that. rather than feel relief when the weight of his arm lifted, she felt its absence said more than she wanted it to say. And she needed to try to get back her certainty that their case was hopeless. That the split between them was not as easy to suture as their earlier patient's head had been. The wound caused by her and Mack's rift had healed and scarred over. For anything to happen between them—like getting back together—that scar would have to be ripped open and allowed to heal all over again, and the thought of that made her cringe. Because if it had hurt the first time, the second time would be an agony that she wasn't sure she could bear. Especially if it held no certainty that it would stay healed this time.

But one thing at a time. First she had to get through this doctor's appointment, and then she could figure out the rest of it. Until then, she would just rest in the realization that Mack did want to go through this with her. At least for now. And until that changed, it would be enough. She would make sure of it.

CHAPTER EIGHT

MACK LOOKED IN surprise at the paper that Rhett dropped onto his desk. "What's this?"

His brother raised his brows. "I saw the job posting and decided to apply for the job."

"The job posting for the ER position?"

"You're the head of that department, aren't you? I wouldn't be here if I were applying for a job in geriatrics."

Frustration rose up inside of him over the flippant response. Then again, that was kind of what his and Rhett's relationship had come to. A series of sparring matches where no one won and where everyone was left feeling unsatisfied. Leave it to Rhett to come in on the very last day of the job notice and upset the apple cart. The apple cart that Mack had very carefully stacked—in favor of Jack Elliot.

"You're serious about this? I thought you were all about your Grand Prix position."

His brother's expression changed, became

something he would have never expected of his brother: somber…almost sad. "Things change."

Yes they did. He'd seen that firsthand. Maybe that's why Lainey's decision to go to Boston had bothered him so much. That it had seemed more like something his brother would do than the wife he thought he'd known. Or could it be that it wasn't the thing the wife he'd constructed inside of his head would do? Had he tried to make Lainey into someone she wasn't?

That bothered him on a level he hadn't explored. Until this very moment.

But why was it wrong for Rhett…or Lainey, for that matter, to decide that they wanted something different? It might not be the way Mack would have gone about making that kind of decision, but Lainey had done well for herself in Boston. And Rhett had done well in his job at the racetrack. He'd heard his brother's name mentioned in the hallways of the hospital more than once.

Could he envy his brother's spontaneity?

Who knew? But right now, that wasn't the problem in front of him. The problem was that he was evidently going to have two very qualified people vying for the same post.

"Well, thanks for coming in. I need to tell you I have one other applicant—and she's been here for a little while." He paused. "I can't show favoritism, Rhett. I'll need to decide based on a lot of different criteria."

"Yeah. I just heard. All I ask is that you give my application a fair chance."

"I would do that with anyone, Rhett." He tried not to be irritated. But part of it was that he was worried about Lainey's upcoming appointment. "I'll do what I think is best for the hospital."

"Got it." Rhett turned to face the door. "Thanks for at least considering it."

Mack stood up. "Hey, wait."

"What is it?"

He debated, before finally saying, "I wanted to let you know that Lainey is expecting."

His brother turned back toward him. "I didn't realize she was involved with anyone."

Ah…no. "That's not what I mean. She's not involved with anyone."

He realized that didn't sound any better. "The baby is mine."

"Wow! You two are back together? I guess congratulations are in order."

"No. We're not. But I am happy about the baby. So thanks." He shrugged. "Anyway, I'll let you know what I decide."

With that, he wrapped up the conversation, not being entirely happy with how he was ending things. But he could think about that later.

Once his brother was out the door, he blew out a breath and sat back in his chair. The last time he'd talked to Rhett, his brother had mentioned maybe needing a change. But this… Mack couldn't imagine working with his brother, much less having to be his boss. That would go over so very well with Rhett. And on top of it all, he had Jack's application too, and while he hadn't promised her the job, he had to admit he'd made it sound almost like a formality. But the last thing he expected was for Rhett to hand in that paperwork. On day seven, of all things. Not to mention that Lainey had her appointment at the birthing center today and was still none the wiser about why they wanted to see her.

His heart had cramped when she said she was scared. She was an independent woman who made her own decisions and who didn't show her emotions easily. Like the divorce. Those papers had been delivered without fanfare, without shouting matches, without tears. It was simply matter-of-fact. A defense mechanism against her father's machinations. He could see that now.

The fact that she opened up about being worried said that she was more than just concerned. Inside she had to be frantic. He had to admit she wasn't the only one. He might have been shocked and just a little horrified by the news of the pregnancy two short weeks ago, but somehow over the course of putting that baby crib and other furniture together—and he'd finished the job two nights ago, while she was at work—he'd grown to love the little being that they'd created. And if something happened to the baby…or to Lainey…

Nothing's going to happen, Mack. It couldn't. Not when he'd just gotten used to the idea. Not when he was looking forward to seeing Lainey's body change as the baby grew inside her.

Not when he'd told his brother the news.

Wow! You two are back together? He could still hear his brother's voice and the genuine congratulations he'd offered.

Mack only wished it was true.

No. It was too late for that. And his instinct said if this breakup happened once, it would happen again, whether due to her wanting to "explore her options" or some other reason. Right? People who divorced very seldom got back together. Not unless they figured out how to handle whatever conflict had broken them up in the first place. And neither he nor Lainey seemed interested in tackling the sore subject of Boston or how they had let themselves get to the point of not talking and allowing the schism between them to become so deep that there'd been no crossing back.

So he would be happy with being able to share this baby with her. At least something good would have come out of their marriage… out of that night of intoxicated lovemaking. And he had to admit it had been intoxicating on more than one level. Because he still remembered enough to set his body on fire and to haunt his dreams deep into the night.

He glanced at his watch. He had a few more minutes before he met her downstairs. They were going to drive together this time, rather than meet at the clinic. The first concession Lainey had made toward the fact that people were eventually going to find out about the pregnancy. After all, he'd told Rhett just before his brother left his office. Maybe it had been to help relieve the tension that had permeated the space when his brother assured him that he knew what he was doing.

Mack hoped his brother was right. But not only that, he hoped that he himself knew what he was doing when it came to Lainey and the baby. Because if he didn't, it wasn't just Mack who would suffer. It would be Lainey too.

They pulled into the parking lot and Mack turned the car off. "Ready?"

"I'm not sure I can do this. If something's wrong…"

He took her hand and carried it to his mouth, pressing his lips to her palm with a gentleness that made her want to weep. "I'll be right there with you. Together we can get through whatever it is."

"What if he or she is…gone?"

He pulled her toward him, pressing his forehead to hers. "We heard the baby's heartbeat. It was strong and steady. I have to believe that means something."

How often had Lainey laid her head on Mack's chest and heard his heartbeat so strong and steady and thought the same thing? That it had to mean something. How often had she drawn her own strength from that sound?

"I hope so. I haven't felt the baby move yet though."

"You won't feel that until eighteen to twenty-two weeks."

Lainey leaned back in surprise. "You remember that from residency?"

"No. I looked it up on Dr. Google."

Laughter burst from her throat before she could stop it. "How often do we tell people that Dr. Google is not their friend?"

"I didn't say it was a proud moment. I simply admitted that I caved and did it."

This time she didn't chuckle, but she did smile. "Thanks. That makes me feel better though, knowing I won't feel the baby until a little later."

"I'm glad. So we're going in there with open minds, right?"

"I'll try."

"Well, let's get in there then."

They got out of the car, and Mack held her hand as they walked to the door. As they checked in at the registration desk. As they sat in their seats. And for once, Lainey didn't care what anyone thought. She was glad of Mack's support. Of feeling like someone was there for her. Not that her mom and sisters weren't. She finally told Hope and the rest of her sisters about the pregnancy, and although they were ecstatic about having another niece or nephew, a few were concerned about what trying to co-parent might be like for Lainey. But despite those reservations, a few of which she agreed with, they all said they would be up for babysitting duty if she ever needed it. All Lainey needed to do was yell and they would all be there at a moment's notice.

"Alaina? You can come back."

She really did need to tell them they could call her Lainey. Having them use her formal name made this visit sound that much more ominous. And the last thing she needed today was ominous.

There was no weigh-in today, she was simply taken straight back to a room where they sat. And sat. And sat.

It reminded her of the time when she was a child and they'd taken their Yorkshire terrier in to be spayed and her sisters and mom all went in to pick her up at the appointed hour. Except they waited in the waiting room until there were no more people there. Only then did the vet come out and ask them to come to her office. "Where's Penny?" Lainey had asked.

The vet then had to break the terrible news that Penny had died during the procedure. They'd tried to revive her, but nothing had worked. The girls had all broken into sobs, and Lainey remembered even the vet's eyes overflowing with tears. "I'm so sorry, guys. We're going to perform an autopsy, if that's okay."

It turned out Penny lacked a pathway in her liver that would have flushed the anesthesia out of her system. There had been nothing the vet could have done and no way she could have known without very specific testing.

Was that why they were sitting here waiting? Did the doctor have some terrible news to give them?

Tracy Lindhart swept into the room with a

smile, rather than an air of doom. "How are you, Alaina?"

"Please call me Lainey. And I'm okay. But I am a little worried. Is something wrong with the baby?"

Tracy made a note in her chart, probably about the nickname.

"No. Not that we've found. But I forgot to mention during your last visit about some genetic testing we'd like to do to look for any chromosomal abnormalities. Just as a precaution. I'd like to be prepared for any eventuality. And it will help you make decisions about treatment."

"Okay." She relaxed. She'd known this was coming, so it wasn't a surprise. "So there was nothing on the sonogram that raised any alarms?"

"No…" She paused as if unsure what Lainey was asking. "Did I miss something in your family history? Like heart defects or kidney deformities?"

"No. Nothing that I know of. I just thought…" She closed her eyes. "Will it be like this the whole pregnancy? Where every phone call makes me think disaster is looming around the corner?"

Tracy sat down. "Probably. And if the staff has made you feel that way, it's my fault and I apologize. I would rather all news about testing and results come through me, so office staff is told to be vague when pressed. If you are ever alarmed though, please ask for a callback from me or from one of the nurses and we'll be happy to do that."

"Okay, thank you." She finally felt strong enough to let go of Mack's hand, realizing her fingers had become a vice around his.

They talked for a few minutes about the kind of testing that Tracy wanted to do, and Lainey said yes to all of it. She might not make a decision based on test results, but she would at least know what was coming and try to prepare for any eventualities.

Tracy left the room to make arrangements.

"Do you want to stay here for the blood draws?" she asked Mack. "If you need to get back to the hospital, I'll be okay. Thanks though for talking me off the ledge. I was so sure something was terribly wrong."

"No. I'll stay. Besides, we drove here together, remember? I didn't want to worry you even more, but I was just a tad concerned myself."

As soon as the nurse had all the vials of blood she needed, she and Mack were free to go on their way. They picked up ice cream cones at a local shop and walked down the street of downtown Austin. They were still several blocks from the hospital. So they wouldn't walk back. They would drive, instead. But it was nice being out in the sun, even though it still wasn't as hot as it was going to get. That would happen in July or August.

"By the way, Rhett came by my office earlier to apply for that job—the one I almost promised to Jack."

"Wow, that must have been an awkward conversation," she said.

"It wasn't exactly fun. But in the process, I also told him about the pregnancy and the fact that the baby is mine."

She nodded. "It's okay. I didn't expect you to keep it a secret from family. I told my sisters. If you want to tell your dad, you're welcome to."

He stiffened, and even before he said anything, she knew he was not going to tell his father. And that made her sad.

"I don't think so. My dad and I haven't spoken in probably a year. And I'm not too thrilled about changing that."

If her dad were still alive, would she have told him? Yes. Because although they didn't have the best relationship, he would have been happy about the news. Was there a reason to think that Thom wouldn't be happy?

She had no idea.

They finished their ice cream and headed back to the car. When they got there, she said, "I'm sorry I brought up your dad."

With his hand on the passenger door handle, he paused. Then he turned. "Lainey, you didn't do anything wrong. I promise." He turned around and leaned his backside on the car door before brushing her hair back from her cheeks. "My dad and I just…"

"I get it. I feel the same way about my father. Sometimes I think it's easier, him being gone. And then I feel such guilt over thinking that."

Gripping her hips, he eased her toward him. "Oh, honey. What is it with us and relationships?"

She leaned against him, elbows in and hands splayed across his chest. The sheer comfort she felt from being physically connected with him was alarming. And yet she didn't want to move away. Couldn't make herself. "I've thought the same thing."

He smiled. "And yet we did at least one thing right."

"Yes we did." The memories of that night flooded back to her. It had been good. So, so good. And there were no regrets. Or at least none that she could think of right now.

And when he tipped her forward and captured her lips in a kiss, she was more than happy to stay right where she was. It started off soft and undemanding. Sweet. Surrounded by the same warm comfort she'd found against his chest. Until she shifted. Frowned. Wanted more than just comfort. If he was going to kiss her, she wanted him to *really* kiss her. She pressed closer.

"Lainey," he whispered against her mouth. "What are you doing to me?"

"The same thing you're doing to me. The thing I *want* you to do to me."

She leaned her cheek against him and inhaled his scent. That familiar smell that tickled her nose and drew her to him.

And right now, she did want him. And she didn't care about their past or their future. She just wanted to feel him against her.

"Get in the car," he murmured. "This venue is just a little too public for me."

She realized they were parked on the street and people were walking by, several of them smiling as they looked their way.

He was right. This was just a little too public.

They got in the car, and when he started the engine, he looked at her. "Tell me where we're going."

She had a feeling if she said the hospital, they would go there and he would drop her off next to her car and that would be that.

But it's not what she wanted.

"Let's go to my place." She didn't want to see where he lived now, having a feeling it would be too sad and would ruin the mood. At least for her. But if they wound up at her apartment, there would be a sense of expectation in the air, still left over from putting the baby furniture together. It seemed right to go there.

"Okay. We'll be there in about ten minutes."

True to his word, it didn't take long for him to find the back streets and intersections that would take them to her apartment complex.

He remembered the number of her spot and parked in one of the spaces assigned to her. "How did you remember?"

"I remember a lot about you. I always did."

Like the fact that she was so quick to take a job that would take her miles and miles away from him? Like the fact that she'd been the one to file for divorce and not him?

But she knew that wasn't what he was talking about. He was talking about her preferences during sex. About what she loved him to do and the things she didn't care for as much.

And that made her feel cared for just like when he'd held her hand when she was afraid the baby had died.

She got out of the car and just then noted a plume of smoke coming from the far side of the second set of apartment complexes. It was too big to be coming from one of the barbecue pits. "Mack, look."

She pointed to the smoke. "I think there's a fire in one of the units."

"Call 911."

While she called, Mack quickly reversed the car and drove in the direction of the smoke. As they pulled up, it was eerily quiet. How could it be that no one had noticed it yet? But then again, it was the middle of the day and most people were at work.

"What's your emergency?"

"There's a fire at the Austin Center Landing Apartments. Unit D. It looks to be apartment 201. There is smoke coming out of one of the windows. I'm at the scene with another doctor."

"Got it. Fire and rescue is en route. Don't attempt to go in on your own."

The sound of screaming suddenly came from the apartment. "Please hurry. I can hear people yelling inside."

"They're five minutes out."

Lainey pressed End, as there was nothing more she could add, and she jumped out of the car.

Mack grabbed her arm before she could charge up the stairs. "Wait. If you go up there, you could make it worse."

"Worse than someone being burned alive?"

"No, but opening that door without knowing what you're doing could result in a flashback and make the fire flare up. We'll help. I promise. As soon as they get here."

Standing there doing nothing was one of the worst things she'd ever felt, even though she knew he was right. Within another minute she heard the sound of sirens headed their way. They stood on the sidewalk, joined by a couple of other people who had also seen the smoke. The firefighters leaped out of the truck and immediately hooked up to a nearby fire hydrant.

Mack went over to let one of them know they were both doctors from Austin Memorial and were standing by to help.

"Great, I'm the fire chief. We'll let you know as soon as we can tell the extent of the fire and locate any survivors."

Survivors. Lainey heard the word over and over in her head. The screaming had stopped. What if whoever belonged to that cry for help had died? "We did hear someone yelling, but without knowing the best way to get to them…"

"You absolutely did right by not trying to go in on your own or we might have had more folks to rescue. Stay close by if you don't mind. I'll be back in a few minutes. EMTs are en route as well."

The chief went off to join the rest of his crew, who were already on the boom lift and shooting water through a second-floor window. Another two firefighters were just now entering the apartment. She sent up a quick prayer.

Mack shot her a glance. "What if you and the baby were in this building? Or worse, in that apartment."

Was he taking a shot at where she'd chosen to live? She'd checked the reviews of Austin Central Landing and the ratings were excellent. And from what she'd seen everything was kept up well. The one time she'd had something happen, maintenance had been over within a half hour and dealt with the problem.

"Fire can break out anywhere. Our old house could have burned down just as easily."

He gripped her hand. "Sorry, Lainey, I'm not criticizing. I just wonder if a house wouldn't be better at some point."

"Um… I'm not thinking about buying a house or getting anything more permanent. Right now, I'm happy where I'm at."

She knew she was being stubborn, but dammit, she wanted to make her own decisions. She was just as capable as he was about thinking things through, although maybe it didn't look like that through his eyes.

The chief came over to them. "We've got two

victims. Both alive, but they're in bad shape. Burns and smoke inhalation. EMTs are just pulling onto the scene, but they can only do so much."

In other words, he wasn't sure they'd make it to the hospital. With the fire chief leading the way, both she and Mack hurried behind him. Lainey was going over protocols for burn victims. Their best bet was to transport as soon as possible, but if either of them were in respiratory or cardiac arrest, they needed to start treatment on the ground. The apartments weren't far from Austin M, so ground transport would be just as fast as calling for Care Flight.

It was a mom and infant. Lainey's heart reacted before she had a chance to tuck it behind her doctor persona. But somehow she managed.

The chief said, "Looks like mom lay over her baby in an attempt to shield her from the fire."

The clothes were singed, and it was hard to tell where the woman's shirt ended and her skin began. "You take the baby," she said. "I'll take Mom."

Lainey wasn't sure she had it in her to turn away from the person who had tried to save her own child. "Any idea what her name is?"

"Apartment manager said it's Theresa Laurence. She's a single mom."

Lainey leaned down, aware that one of the EMT workers had knelt beside her.

"Theresa, can you hear me?"

She lifted her head and her eyes fluttered, arms waving. "M-my baby."

"We're helping your baby right now. But we need to check you over."

Just then the woman's head fell back, eyes rolling in her head. Lainey grabbed the woman's hand, feeling for a pulse. Nothing. "Check for a heartbeat?"

The paramedic put his stethoscope to her burned chest and shook his head. "She's in cardiac arrest."

"Get a blanket under her back."

They quickly put a blanket over the mulch and turned her onto her back. Lainey started compressions while the first responder got a portable defibrillator out and ready.

"Keep going. I'm going to work around you," he said.

Lainey nodded but didn't stop chest compressions while he put one of the pads on the right side of Theresa's chest and one on the lower left side. The shock would need to go through the patient's chest cavity to have the best chance of restarting the heart.

"Stop compressions."

Lainey leaned back so that her body wasn't in contact with the patient's. The defibrillator's mechanical voice notified them that it was analyzing the heartbeat. When it couldn't find one it stated that it was charging the system. "All clear."

The defibrillator sent a charge through the patient, and her body contracted. The heartbeat was analyzed again. Shocked again. Still nothing.

Lainey resumed compressions. "Let's get epinephrine on board."

"Start an IV or intraosseous?"

"Intraosseous. Let's do proximal tibia." It might be difficult to find a vein, considering the severe burns she had on so much of her body.

She was so focused on her own patient that she'd zoned out everything else until she heard the cry of a baby. She faltered for a split second before she continued with renewed vigor. "Come on, Mama. Don't you give up on me."

Lainey was aware of the paramedic clearing clothing and sanitizing the skin before using the large bore needle and driving it into the bone, drawing up a little marrow to make sure he was in position. Then he administered the drug.

"Let's switch," he said.

The paramedic moved to Lainey's spot to

continue compressions while she monitored for a pulse. Two minutes after the epinephrine had been administered, she got something.

“Stop. We have a pulse. It’s thready, but there.”

The emergency responder said, “Let’s get her transported while we can.” He turned to his partner, who was helping with the baby. “How are you coming?”

“We can go at any time. The baby is stable.”

Thank God. She only hoped Theresa held on until they got to the hospital. With oxygen masks in place, they loaded both patients into the truck, giving Lainey and Mack a wave before they closed the back doors of the vehicle and took off in the direction of Austin M, sirens blaring.

The firefighters had succeeded in extinguishing the fire, and what Lainey hadn’t realized as they were fighting to save Theresa’s life was that the rest of that block of apartments had been evacuated and people were standing around, some crying.

As her adrenaline levels bottomed out, Lainey had to fight her own emotions. She hoped they made it. Turning to Mack, she whispered, “Can we go to the hospital?”

He took hold of her arm and turned her to face him. “Are you feeling okay?”

Realizing he was worried about her own health, she nodded. “I’m fine. But… I have to know.”

He nodded. “I was thinking the same thing. Let’s go.”

CHAPTER NINE

THEY GOT TO the hospital a few minutes after the paramedics, and Mack didn't stop to think what they must look like. He glanced at Lainey to see that her white blouse was dirty and she had dark smears and a smudge across one cheek—all from the charring from the fire. Her hair gave evidence of the heat of the day and working on her burn victim, hanging in moist strands around her face and down her back. Despite all of that, she was beautiful. Even more so for how hard she had worked to save Theresa. He'd thought he'd handed her the easier of the two cases when they were first brought out of the building, but the baby had been relatively stable, with few burns thanks to his mother's quick thinking.

He realized that, while they knew Theresa's name, she hadn't been conscious enough to tell them the baby's name, so the paramedic had just written down Baby Doe. They figured they could get a name later.

The paramedics were still in the ER, filling in the staff at the reception desk with what they knew about the patients. Daphne, who'd just come out from the back, saw them.

"Oh my God, what happened?"

The paramedic who'd been working with Lainey glanced over and then made his way toward them. "These two were on the scene and helped with the patients." He held his hand out. "I don't think we were introduced. I'm Abe Matthews and my partner is Rick Sanchez."

He shook both their hands, lingering just a touch longer over Lainey's as they both introduced themselves. Mack couldn't hold back a slight frown.

"Nice to finally have names." He smiled. "Thanks for pitching in today."

"How are they?" Lainey's voice was quiet as if she wasn't sure she wanted to know.

"Theresa stabilized en route, surprising us both." Something about the way he said it made Mack take a closer look at him.

In the meantime, Lainey's eyes closed, and he could hear her breathe, "Thank God."

Mack waited a second or two before asking the obvious question. "The baby?"

"He seemed okay, when we loaded up. He

was responsive and struggling to cry, but then his oxygen levels plummeted and he went into respiratory arrest. They're working on him right now."

Lainey's eyes widened. "Oh no!"

They both knew it could happen. Smoke inhalation could seem innocuous at first, but could cause inflammation that ultimately led to respiratory collapse.

His partner came over and clapped him on the back. "We need to go. Chief is saying that we might be needed back at the scene for a possible heart attack."

Abe gave them a quick wave and then headed out with his partner. They both seemed so young. So full of life and able to brush off what had happened. Mack knew it was a defense mechanism and something they and all medical staff were trained to do, but today he just wasn't feeling it. And if Lainey's face were any indication, she wasn't either.

"Do you want to wait?"

"Yes," she said. "Could we? I just need to know."

"I get it." He felt the same. But if she'd wanted to leave he would have followed her home, since her car was still parked at the hospital.

Her doctor's appointment seemed so long ago

now. Like it had happened in a different lifetime. Thank God it hadn't been bad news. Because having the burn victims stacked on top of it would have been hard. Too hard.

"Let's go get a cup of coffee."

They headed down the hallway, and Mack halted in his tracks. Lainey looked at him and her head tilted. "What is it?"

"Look."

Rhett and Jack Elliot were standing in front of the café, and it looked like they were having a heated discussion. Did these two know each other?

It sure seemed that way. Could it be about the position?

Maybe he needed to intervene. He glanced down at Lainey. "Do you mind going in the café first when we get closer, and I'll meet you in there in a few minutes?"

"Of course. Are you going to talk to them?"

"I'm going to make sure things are okay."

Just before they got to the café, Jack and Rhett noticed them and went silent. Jack at least attempted a greeting, but Rhett's eyes were on Mack as if he'd created the problem. He hadn't. And he wasn't exactly sure how to solve it, but maybe he could serve as some kind of a buffer.

Lainey ducked into the establishment with

a hushed greeting for both of them, and then left Mack to talk to them.

She ordered both their coffees, since she knew that Mack took his black. Then she found a table and waited.

Lainey had half expected to get to the hospital and find out that Theresa had crashed again, and with the extent of her burns, even if she pulled through this initial stage, there was always the danger of infection setting in and making her take another turn for the worse. And then there would be countless skin grafts and plastic surgeries, although since her face had been over her baby, the skin there looked intact. The worst of it was on her back and arms with some singed areas on her chest. The polyester in her shirt had melted and was stuck to her, and removing it was going to be a painful process.

But if her baby died, it might take away her reason for living, since it looked like this was her only child, and the firefighters said she was a single mom.

She wanted them both to make it in a way that went beyond the doctor/patient relationship. Maybe it was because of her own baby tucked safely in her womb. Putting herself in Theresa's place, how would she deal with things? If Mack were involved in the baby's life, she wouldn't technically be a single mom, right? He wouldn't be living with her, but he would be around.

And if a fire had broken out in her apartment and Mack hadn't been there? It was doubtful that he would be in the space even 30 percent of the time. His comment about the complex was probably in reference to that. That he'd been worried about something happening and him not being around.

But he wouldn't be. Unless they got back together. And it didn't look like that was going to happen. Despite how right it had felt to have him putting together baby furniture in her apartment those two days. She'd allowed herself to fantasize about…

Mack appeared and her thoughts went up in smoke.

She cringed at that thought and did her best to shake it off. "How did things go?"

"As well as they could have." He shrugged. "They were talking about the position. But there's nothing I can do about that. They'll have to figure it out."

He sat down, and she pushed his cup of coffee toward him. "Thanks."

Lainey glanced at him. Despite what they'd

been through at the apartment complex, he looked good. So very good. And she…

She had to look a mess, and her hair felt stuck to the back of her neck in a way that made her wrinkle her nose. Pulling a clip out of her purse, she twisted her hair and put it up, the cool of the air conditioner curling around her nape making her feel a hundred times better.

“I’ll be right back,” Mack said.

He got a bottle of water and paid for it and then returned to the table.

“Sorry,” Lainey said. “I didn’t even think about—”

“It’s not for me.” He opened the bottle and poured a little bit onto a napkin. “Give me your arm.”

She glanced down and realized her shirt was dirty and that soot was smeared all over her right arm. Probably because her left hand had been in contact with Theresa’s clothing and skin while doing chest compressions. She’d then transferred it to other places on her body and clothing.

“It’s okay, I can…”

He took her arm and gently swiped the cool cloth over her skin, wiping away some of the dirt. Her emotions went all wonky and she thought about how this would have been something she wouldn’t have thought twice about back when they were together. How many times had they soaped each other up in the shower? How often had she smeared dirt on his face as they worked in the garden of their home?

It was something that had seemed so natural back then. But now?

It had to be the baby hormones. Because the same emotions she'd felt as she'd watched him put furniture together were back in full force.

He finished cleaning her arm and then got a fresh napkin and added more water. Then he leaned forward. When she pulled her head away, not sure what he was planning to do, he murmured, "Trust me, Lainey."

She did. She always had. It was Mack who'd had the trust issues in their marriage. Yes, she'd bristled when he suggested how to do things or gave her unwanted advice, but she'd never stopped trusting him. Until he refused to move to Boston with her.

And when she looked back, she wasn't quite sure if Boston had been about career opportunities or if she'd felt pushed into it by him questioning if it was a wise thing to do.

Plus they'd been trying to have a baby for six months, and the job offer had come just as she'd unexpectedly gotten her period when she had hoped beyond hope that that would be the month. Maybe she'd been fleeing what she viewed as failure and had felt like she needed a change of scenery. Could it be that deep down she'd known he wouldn't come and it was her way of running away from her life? Somewhere he wasn't likely to follow her.

And the divorce?

Oh yes, that had been about his lack of communication, and she'd felt like he hadn't cared that she was gone. Then her head started messing with her even further, making her wonder if he was secretly glad she'd left. Filing papers had been a test. One neither one of them had passed.

And they'd never really talked about any of it. Even after she'd come back to Austin and told him she was pregnant.

Then the rental apartment? And the papers on her dining room table? Were those contingency plans in case things didn't work out?

Probably.

The second he touched her face though, dabbing away whatever was on it, she started having second thoughts. Could she really leave him again?

She didn't think so.

Her eyes met his, and there was something warm and soft in his glance. Something she hadn't seen since… Since they started trying to get pregnant. Things had turned mechanical and cold-bloodedly planned during that time. The warmth in his gaze had cooled, and although the sex was still so, so good, it wasn't the same. And she'd missed that closeness, even as she started to chafe against all the other stuff.

"Thank you, Mack."

He drew the moist cloth down the bridge of her nose, making her smile.

"My pleasure," he said.

And those words. The gruffness of them. The way they could be taken so differently from the situation at hand…

She wanted to be with him. Wanted him to love her the way she…

The way she still loved him.

And she realized she did. She still loved him. She'd never stopped, even after the separation and the anger and the signing of papers. That night in Boston should have told her that. But maybe she hadn't been ready to listen to her heart back then.

But she was ready to now. Could he trust her the way she trusted him?

She didn't know. But something in her hoped so.

Daphne appeared in the doorway of the café and motioned to them.

Her face was serious, and Lainey immediately knew it was bad news. God, she'd been sitting here dreaming of a future with Mack and had almost forgotten that Theresa and her baby were in this very hospital fighting for their lives.

At least she hoped they were still alive, even if things weren't looking good.

She got up from the table, and they followed Daphne back to the ER. "Dr. Jones wants to talk to you both."

Okay, maybe it wasn't horrific news if the retiring doctor wanted to update them in person. Someone had probably told him that she and Mack had been on the scene and had rendered first aid.

"He's in the back."

"Thanks," Lainey said.

She and Mack went through the doors, while Daphne went back to her triage area. Dr. Jones was waiting for them in the hallway. That was odd; she would have expected Theresa and her baby to have already had several specialists swarming them, each trying to help fix different areas of their patients.

Carter leaned a shoulder against a nearby wall as if needing the support. He looked older than his years right now, and a chill went over her. "I thought you both deserved an update."

"Thanks," Mack said. "How are they?"

"Theresa is back getting tests run, and if we

can keep her stable, they'll start the process of debriding some of her burns and trying to remove the clothing that has fused with her skin."

"And the baby?" This time Lainey asked the question, but she was pretty sure she didn't want to know the answer.

Carter shook his head. "He didn't make it. His lungs started filling with fluid from the inflammation and we couldn't keep up with it. They told you he crashed on the way in?"

Her heart spasmed, and she couldn't see clear to even answer.

Mack answered for her. "The paramedics told us."

"We never got him back. But by God, we did our damnedest. I swear we did."

The old ER doctor never said the normal platitudes about the baby having gone peacefully, because the ER was not a place of peace. It was a war zone where every foot gained came with a struggle that most people rarely ever witnessed other than those who were involved in the fight. She could only imagine what the room where that baby was treated looked like.

On second thought, she didn't want to imagine it. Because she'd seen it time and time again. And somehow she'd gotten through it. Often there'd been a sense of sorrow at another battle loss, but it had to be pushed aside as there was always another patient, always another fight to try to win.

Carter knew that. When she looked in his eyes, she knew that's why he needed the support that the wall next to him offered. And probably why he was retiring at just fifty-five years of age. He was tired of losing this particular fight.

She couldn't blame him. She was suddenly tired of it too. All of it. Maybe she'd been wrong to leave Boston. At least in administration, she didn't see as much of this side of ER life. And yes, she'd missed it. But not this. Never this.

Before she could stop them, the tears came. It wasn't Mack who enfolded her in his arms though. It was the wizened doctor, who left his perch and held her while she cried. And cried.

"I know," he said. "Believe me, I know."

When the sobs finally slowed, she leaned back, sniffling. "Has Theresa been told?"

"Not yet. We want to give her some time. We'll clean Bradley up and dress him. If Theresa is able to, in the next twenty-four or forty-eight hours, we'll put him in a cuddle cot and let her say her goodbyes."

Bradley. His name had been Bradley. Somehow it helped knowing, although she wasn't sure why. And she was so glad they were going to try to use a cuddle cot with him.

Looking much like a normal bassinet, the specialized cots were often used for stillborn babies to give the parents a chance to say their goodbyes. The cooling feature helped preserve the body, and could be used for up to seventy-two hours. At least that's what she remembered during her maternity rotation.

It could help relatives process the death.

But it wouldn't change the reality.

She eased away from Carter, wiping her eyes. "Sorry for the waterworks."

"Don't be. I don't think there was a dry eye in that room when we finally called it."

"Thank you for trying."

He nodded. "Thank you for trying on the scene. I hear that Theresa might not have stood a chance if you hadn't been there."

"She wanted to live. I hope she continues to want that."

She didn't have to say what she meant. But when she glanced at Mack, he was looking over their heads as if only half listening. Suddenly she knew why he hadn't been the one to hug her. He'd commented on how that could have been her and the baby when they'd arrived on the scene. Whereas she'd taken it as criticism, maybe he'd simply been imagining the unimaginable.

"Thanks again, Carter."

He took one last look at them and nodded, heading back into the bowels of the department, probably headed for another room…another patient…and another battle. She hoped the rest of today was better than this moment had been.

Once he was out of sight, she glanced at Mack, then turned and put her arms around his waist, laying her head on his chest, not caring who might happen upon them.

"Can we get out of here? Please?" she asked.

"Yes."

Stepping back, she started to move ahead of him to lead the way, only to have him reach down and grip her hand instead. And hand in hand they walked back through the doors of the ER. They passed Daphne on the way out, and Lainey was pretty sure she saw the other woman's lips curve in the semblance of a smile.

CHAPTER TEN

As IF BY unspoken agreement, they didn't stop in the parking lot to get Lainey's car, and instead he opened his car door for her and got into the driver's seat. He glanced at her, and when she held out her hand, palm side up, he took hold of it again, just like he'd done on the way out of the hospital.

He couldn't believe the baby hadn't made it, although he'd seen enough cases that he knew things could change at a moment's notice. He'd seen it time and time again. Sometimes that change worked in their favor, and sometimes it didn't. All he knew right now was that he was glad for this physical connection to Lainey. Glad that she seemed to want that human touch too. He should have been the one to hold her in the ER, but he'd been picturing another very different scene. One where it was Lainey and her baby lying on that ground. One where his baby had died instead of Theresa's. And he hadn't been able to process it. So instead he'd tuned everything out, until Lainey had turned to him—very much alive.

He was so incredibly grateful. All the stupid stuff that had happened between them seemed to melt away. He lifted her hand to his lips and kissed the backs of her fingers.

When they got to her place, they sat in the car for a minute or two trying to ignore the singed building on the other side of the lot.

She turned to him. "Please come in, Mack." Her fingers reached up to touch his face. "Please. I just need you to hold me."

He didn't say anything because the words were all clogged in his throat. He needed that too. Needed to hold her and be held by her.

She unlocked the door and let him go in ahead of her before closing it behind them. She tossed her keys onto the small table in the foyer and then took his hands and faced him. Going up on tiptoe, she tried to reach his face and was just a little too short, so he bent down to peck her on the cheek. But she turned her face at the last second so that her mouth met his.

And then all bets were off. He just needed to know she was here. Alive. And with him. A huge wave of need washed over him, and he picked her up in his arms and headed for the couch, tossing her on its long length before following her down. When he settled against her, he felt like he'd come home after a long absence and found a familiar welcome. One he'd missed so very much.

"Lainey..." He muttered her name against her mouth, only to have her silence whatever he'd been going to say by wrapping her arms around his neck and pulling him closer, opening her mouth to him.

And suddenly talking didn't matter. Talking could wait. Right now he needed her, and it looked like she needed him just as much.

He pushed her shirt up and kissed her belly, the slight smell of smoke from the fire reaching his nose. No. Not like this. The last thing he needed was a reminder of what they'd just been through. He hefted himself from her and stood, but when she whimpered and held her arms out to him, he took her hand and hauled her up to stand by him. "Come on, I have an idea."

He knew her bathroom was in between the two bedrooms and he found it, quickly pushing the door shut with his foot and turning on the taps in her bathtub, which looked like it was just the right size...

And while it was filling, he turned toward her and took hold of the bottom of her white tank top and pulled it over her head. Her shirt must have had a bra built into it because there was nothing under there but bare breasts, and staring at them, he dumped the garment into the small hamper that was open against the wall beside her. Then his own shirt came off. When he reached for the button of her jeans and opened it and guided the zipper slowly down, he noticed the slight convexity of her belly. His palm glided over it and stopped there. When he looked in her face, her eyes were closed, lips parted as she breathed.

The woman was gorgeous. So breathtakingly beautiful. He stepped forward, trapping her between him and the bathroom vanity, and then reached behind her to set her hair free from her clip, tossing it onto the countertop where a curling iron sat. Then his hands slid down her bare back, relishing the soft skin under his palms. He continued on until he reached the waistband of her jeans and dipped just below the barrier. When the countertop interfered with his journey, he tugged her far enough away that he could continue, cupping the curves of that glorious ass that he remembered so well.

"Mack…the tub."

At first he thought she was saying that she wanted to continue this in the bathtub, but no, he'd forgotten he left the water running and it was getting close to being full. He turned off the taps and then came back to kiss her deeply. "Are you sure about this?"

She smiled. "Do I seem sure?" She then unzipped his jeans, sliding in and freeing him. Her fingers wrapped around him and squeezed, making him shudder.

"Yes, you do." He growled the words and then grabbed her wrist, pulling it free. "But it's been a while and I want this to…" He kissed her, punctuating his next words with tiny touches of his lips. "To. Last."

They finished undressing and he stepped into the tub, glad that the water temperature seemed to be just perfect. Then he held out his hand and she joined him. This time when his hands found her butt, one of them glided over and around until he reached the spot where he soon hoped to be. There was a moist heat, and memories surfaced of being deep inside of her. He suddenly wanted to rush and grab at all of it. But he also knew he'd spoken the truth. This time would be different than Boston. Because he would hold himself back. He would hold her back.

Probing the opening, his slid his middle finger inside, her breathy gasp telling him she too remembered this.

"You're sure the doctor said this was okay?"

He wanted her desperately but also wasn't willing to risk hurting her.

"I didn't ask her, but I did look it up. After we kissed that time."

She'd been thinking about this for all that time? Lainey wasn't the only one. Actually, he'd been thinking about it since they'd spent those hours together in Boston, only for him to wake up the next day to find she'd left without a word.

No. Don't think about that. Relish the feel of her under your hands. The way you're going to feel as you slide deep into her.

He let go of her, took hold of the shower wand, removed it from the spot on the wall and let it disappear beneath the surface. Mack was going to need that in a minute. Then he sank down into the warm water, reaching his hands up for her so she would do the same. He put his legs on either side of her hips and crooked his knees so that the soles of her feet were against him, then he pulled her forward. Finding a bottle of her shampoo behind his left arm, he urged her to lie back so that he could wet her hair. She did, and her long hair slid beneath the surface of the water as he carefully leaned over her and cupped her head so that he could control it and made sure every strand was wet. His other hand slid down her belly and over her mound, but when she went to push up into him, he shook his head. "Not yet, baby. Let's get you soaped up."

He sat her back upright, her hair streaming water down her back. Then he opened her bottle of shampoo, a familiar scent wrapping around him as he squirted a small amount into his hand. He gently massaged it into her scalp, letting the smell of honeysuckle envelop him. He used the same shampoo to wash her, letting his hands glide the stuff over her. He was sure she had body soap, but did it really matter? And from the low sounds coming from her, she didn't really care about technicalities either.

He reached around her to turn on the taps and adjusted the temperature and then used the sprayer to rinse her off, quickly washing his own hair and body too. Then he opened the plug in the bottom of the tub just enough to keep up with the flow of the incoming water.

"Turn around the other way, honey."

She frowned at him but did as he asked. "Trust me?"

"Yes." The word was whispered as if she were anticipating something good was coming down the pike. It was. He knew how much she liked this.

He pulled her tight against him, so that he

was trapped between his belly and her back, his own need ramping up more and more by the second. Then he took the shower wand and aimed it toward the front of her, letting the spray run over her neck, over her chest and over her breasts, the hiss of air saying she did indeed remember this. He glanced at the wand and saw it had different options, so he set it for the massage feature, and the gentle spray changed into a pulsed stream and release rhythm that did as much for his libido as it would do for her, even though he wasn't the one experiencing it. Except for vicariously. And that in and of itself was pretty heady.

She moaned when the new, more-directed water hit her sensitive nipples, and Mack's palm curved over one of her breasts while he let the water lave over her other one. He allowed it to stay there for a few seconds until her hand directed it away as if it were too intense. Except then, she pushed his hand lower and he knew what she wanted.

"That is so hot, babe." Keeping his hand on the wand, he waited for her to move it. "Show me."

When her fingers curled over his, she edged his hand down, having no problem sending the stream over her stomach as it headed ever downward in a slow arc.

Still pressed against her back, his flesh leaped, wanting something that wasn't available to him. Yet.

Still she moved down, and Mack rested his chin on her right shoulder. Pausing periodically to kiss her neck, sucking once on the sensitive skin he found there. Later he would allow himself the luxury of a more in-depth exploration, because he was determined that this was not going to be the only time they came together tonight. The shower wand dipped below the surface of the water and continued to slide farther into the depths. The angle changed, as she guided his hand more toward the center and curved the spray just so. Then she tensed, her head falling against his chest as his free hand trapped her nipple between his thumb and forefinger and raised it to a strong peak.

She moaned and her hips began looking for something. Something that wasn't there yet.

Soon, honey. It's coming soon.

His hand left her breast and wrapped around her waist, pulling her tight against him as he continued to allow her to direct the spray of water to where she wanted it.

"Mack..."

His lips went to her ear, biting at her lobe,

needing her like he'd never needed anyone in his life. This woman had always done it for him. She was the only one who ever had.

Suddenly she cried out, her thrusts becoming wild and uncontrolled, and she let go of his hand. "I need… I need…"

He knew exactly what she needed. He hauled her up to her knees and came up behind her, entering her with a controlled thrust.

Hell, he wanted her so bad. Didn't want to hurt her. Didn't want to do something he shouldn't. So he shortened his movements as much as he could until she tilted her head back. "Go, Mack. It's okay, I promise." She huffed out a breath. "I promise…"

The words tore the control from him, and he pumped into her in an old familiar rhythm that they both knew so well.

"Yessssss." The single word told him all he needed to know. She liked it.

Before he could stop it, he reached his climax in a rush, bending her forward at the waist and thrusting out his release until he was spent. Then he eased her back, wrapping his arms around her and letting her lie against him. He closed his eyes, letting the tiny spurts of pleasure continue to periodically radiate through him, until she whispered his name.

"Mmm?"

She turned around to face him and kissed his mouth. "Unless you want to turn into a block of ice, we'd better get out of here. The hot water is all gone."

He realized he'd left the water on and had simply dropped the thing into the tub when they'd come together. But she was right. The water was rapidly cooling.

"Hell. Sorry." He reached forward and switched off the water.

She laughed. "Don't be. I'm not. It was worth it."

"Was it?" He said the words against her mouth.

"Definitely." She paused and looked at him for a minute. "Care to share my bed with me?"

He smiled. "I thought you'd never ask."

Mack hauled her up and out of the tub and used a towel to dry her off and then himself. Then he discarded it onto the ground, and they went hand in hand into her room and shut the door.

Lainey woke up in a haze of happiness and crazy satiation that made it hard for her to move. She smiled and turned her head to the side, expecting to see him sleeping beside her. After all, they hadn't actually curled up together to sleep until just before daylight. Neither one of them had said the words, but she put all the love she could feel into her lovemaking, hoping he would understand the way he used to, when they had been tuned into the other's thoughts and emotions.

And she was pretty sure she sensed what she was feeling in his lovemaking as well. At least she hoped it meant what she thought it did. That he still loved her too. She would ask him straight out this morning.

Except he wasn't in bed with her. The indent of his head was still on the pillow and the duvet was turned back, showing where he'd exited the covers. Maybe he was showering.

She fell back onto the pillows. She was never going to look at that shower wand the same way again, without feeling exactly what he'd done with it. Actually, she was the one who'd done it, moving his hand to where she'd wanted it.

Suddenly she wanted him again, despite the fact that they'd made love two more times. She touched her belly and smiled again. "Sorry about the rocking and rolling in there. But Daddy and I needed a little something."

Silence greeted her from her stomach, just like the silence from the room. A trickle of foreboding entered her system. Shouldn't she hear the shower, if he were in there? She'd never had overnight guests in the apartment before, so she wasn't quite sure what she would hear. Or wouldn't hear.

She got up and found a silky bathrobe hanging on the back of her door. She wrapped it around her and tied the waist. Then she ventured into the hallway, listening. Still there was no sound.

Now she was worried. "Mack? Are you here?"

Did he have a shift this morning? Surely he would have mentioned that if so. She didn't have to be in today until noon.

He didn't answer, so he must have left. She went back into the bedroom and glanced at both the nightstands. No note. And when she retrieved her phone from the charger, there were no messages, no missed calls.

Had she misread the signals? Was this Boston all over again?

No. She'd been the one to leave that time. Was he giving her a little taste of her own medicine?

A sour taste entered her mouth, but she shook her head. No, last night had not seemed like revenge sex. At all. It had seemed…genuine. They'd both been totally into the moment. All three times.

She started to press the number listed beside his name, but something made her stop. Venturing into the bathroom, she wasn't surprised to find that his clothes were gone. Hers had all been neatly tossed into the hamper.

Then she went into the living room and the kitchen and found nothing. There were no remnants to suggest he might have eaten anything and the coffee pot was cold, the lid still propped open like it normally was when she left it to dry in the mornings. Mack never did that with the pot. He'd always put it upside down on a towel. She went back into the living room and glanced toward the dining room, and a sense of horror swept through her as she saw the sheaf of papers lying out in the open. She hadn't put away the letters from various hospitals asking her to consider them for her next home.

She'd started getting those right after she turned her resignation in at Boston. She hadn't thought anything about it, but it seemed amusing to have medical centers from all over the country reach out and get in contact with her. When she moved here, she unpacked one of the boxes and had come across the little stack and laid them out to read. It had been kind of heady, and since she'd pretty much taken the job at Austin M right out of medical school, Boston had been the only other hospital she'd ever been at. She'd put them in a little pile on her dining room table. Maybe as a kind of trophy. A reminder that *someone* wanted her, even if Mack didn't.

Why didn't you just throw them away?

Maybe Mack hadn't even seen them. Of course he had. He'd probably gone into the kitchen to make coffee and spotted them.

Or maybe he'd simply had second thoughts and left.

She moved closer and saw that there was a sheet of paper on top of the stack, with a handwritten note on it. And she recognized that lettering.

Mack.

Her heart in her throat, she made her way over there.

She could almost hear his voice as she read the staccato phrases that spelled out a deep hurt.

Didn't realize you were looking. Again.

I need time to think.

I would like to be informed of what this means for my relationship with my child.

You know where to reach me.

Oh, and your car is out front.

She dropped into one of the chairs and stared at the note. To call him right now would probably find her on the receiving end of everything that note hinted at. And more. So she would give him a few days to cool off. Although this felt like an exact repeat of their conversation right before she decided she was definitely taking the job in Boston. There was no hint that he would go with her, if she was looking. There was no comment about wanting to know what this meant for them as a couple, only about what it meant for him. As a father.

Hadn't she had a couple of weird vibes from comments he'd made about the baby? As if he was only accepting her because she was carrying his child. She'd brushed them off at that time. But now…

Well, now she didn't know what to think. So maybe she needed to take some time to think too. If he was only willing to be with her if she promised to never leave Austin, could she do that? She didn't think so. Because that would mean he only wanted life on his terms. And since his relationships with his father and brother were both fractured and he'd never reached out to his half sister, that didn't look very promising for any romantic reunion between her and Mack.

Yes, she needed to think things through. And then she needed to make a decision and stick with it.

CHAPTER ELEVEN

THREE DAYS AFTER he'd left Lainey's apartment, Mack sat in his office but was no longer congratulating himself over the cool and methodical steps he'd taken to remove himself from her life. The way she'd removed herself from his all those years ago. Firstly, he'd left her a note telling her what to expect—unlike when she'd disappeared from his hotel room in Boston. Secondly, he'd gotten her car keys off the table in her foyer and had gone to the hospital and retrieved her little Honda, driving it back to her place so she wouldn't be without transportation, and then Ubered his way back to the hospital. Thirdly, he'd let her know that he was still willing to be part of his child's life, if she would let him know the parameters. Fourthly, he'd told her exactly what he needed from her: time.

He'd wrapped everything up in a neat package. Because the fact was, those letters from several large university hospitals spoke to the reality that she was willing to entertain offers. As long as those offers didn't come from him.

She was willing to leave him all over again, and yet she'd given him no warning. Except, maybe she had. When he mentioned her getting a house, she'd talked about not wanting anything permanent.

Like maybe even in the relationship department.

How stupid had he been to think maybe they really had a chance to start over? He'd acted impulsively, something not like him, and assumed things that weren't in evidence.

But where was she? He knew for a fact that she wasn't off for three days in a row, because she'd never called him to ask for time off. Maybe she'd taken one of those jobs and hadn't bothered to give Austin M notice.

No. Someone would have come and asked him where she was. But no one had. Which was odd.

He did know one person he could call though.

No. He wasn't going to call her. He was going to march over to her office and ask her outright.

All the offices were housed on the second floor. All except for the hospital administrator, whose office needed to be easily accessible to staff and patrons, so she was located on the first floor at the end of the hallway.

He took the elevator down to the ground floor and headed to her office. Fortunately she was in and she was alone.

"Mack, to what do I owe the pleasure?" Her smile wasn't warm, nor was it welcoming. But he wasn't going to let that stop him.

"Did you do some meddling in my department again?"

"I have no idea what you're talking about."

Good thing he and Glenda were friends or this probably wouldn't end well for him. It still might not if he made her angry enough.

"I think you do. I have a doctor who hasn't shown up for three days. Did she quit?"

"I assume you're not talking about Dr. Lacy." She sat up a little straighter. "You've had some staff who haven't exactly been happy recently. First Carter Jones. Then Valerie Lacy. And now Alaina Thornton. Anything you want to share with me?"

He dropped into a chair, his brain trying to fathom what Glenda had just said. "Lainey left?"

"Not entirely. She asked to be allowed to go work at one of the clinics for a while until she decided what to do in the long run."

So she *was* thinking about taking one of those jobs.

"Did she say why?"

"No. And yes, I asked." Glenda put her elbows on her desk and steepled her fingers. "I asked her outright if this had anything to do with you. Do you know what she told me?"

"I assume you're going to let me know."

"She said she was pregnant and that she thought the work at the clinic would be a little less strenuous." She sighed. "Listen, Mack, I don't know what's going on between the two of you, but I have a feeling this all boils down to you. Am I right?"

"Yes." The word was a single miserable syllable that encased everything he was feeling right now.

"You're the father?"

"Yes again, although she didn't want anyone to know that yet. I assume you can keep it quiet."

She nodded. "Of course. What else?"

"It's not my story to tell. But yes, I do think she left because of me. But I wish you would have talked to me before making the decision to allow her to go."

Her head tilted and she gave him a challenging glance. "I'm still the hospital administrator. After Valerie turned in her notice, I know Dr.

Elliot approached you about the job. I encouraged you to hire her but reminded you that you had to put up a job notice. But suddenly I hear you're letting your brother work here too, effectively replacing one outgoing doctor with two replacements. That leaves us one salary over budget. So I let Lainey go to the clinic. That puts us back on budget. We have Carter Jones's position and Valerie Lacy's filled."

"Rhett and Jack both working was supposed to be a temporary measure until I could decide which one of them stays permanently."

"Well, when you decide that, I'll call Lainey home. If she wants to come back, that is." She shot him a glance. "I expect you to make this right, whatever it is."

His mouth tightened. "I can't guarantee she's going to stay long-term."

"Any proof you can give me of that?"

He wasn't willing to let Glenda know what he'd found. "No."

"Well, I can't guarantee any of us are going to stay long-term. You included." She smiled, and he took that to mean her words weren't a threat.

"True." He shrugged. "I'll make a decision on Rhett and Jack soon."

"Good. And you'll want to bring Lainey back?"

He nodded. "If she wants to come back."

"And if she doesn't?" She shook her head. "Never mind. We can decide that when the time comes. And now…" She waved her hand over her desk as if showing him the piles of tasks she had left to do.

"I can take a hint."

"Can you, Mack? I would have never said you were a stupid individual, but I'm beginning to wonder."

He nodded. "I know. You're not the only one."

Because he was beginning to wonder that about himself. But he had no idea how to make things right, or at this point if that was even possible.

Lainey was surprised at how busy the clinic was. Sofie hadn't been kidding when she'd said they could use more help. But at least she was not having to see Mack each and every day. Because she wasn't sure what to say to him or if there was even anything she could say. It seemed he had laid out his intentions pretty clearly. And if she decided to change jobs again, he would not go with her this time either. He would just let her go.

And since he hadn't tried to call her even after three days of not being at the main hospital, it seemed he really didn't care whether she stayed or went. As to what he'd said about the baby…wouldn't he want to settle that? Or was it going to be the same thing? If the baby wasn't right here where he could have access, would he simply ghost her and his child? There was no way she would allow that. And at some point she was going to have to make that clear. Before the baby was born.

Glenda had said the position here at the clinic was open-ended. She could come back whenever she wanted. But she also said she was not going to let Mack know that. She was going to use this opportunity to teach him a little lesson. Lainey had cringed when the administrator said that. Glenda's lessons were known for being stinging reminders of who was in charge if someone crossed her. And evidently she was feeling protective of Lainey, even though she didn't need protecting. What she had been appreciative of, though, was having a buffer between her and her ex. At least until she decided to tackle this head-on. She just hadn't felt the time was right yet. But it soon would be.

Mack came out of an exam room after treating a patient with whiplash from being dragged by a Newfoundland who'd seen a rabbit and had torn off after it. He never would have guessed it possible, but evidently it was. He prescribed a neck brace and recommended obedience classes. The lady laughed. "For me or my dog?" she'd asked.

Well, at least someone got a good laugh out of it. Mack wasn't laughing at much of anything these days.

Just then the double doors at the entrance to the ER opened and EMTs raced into the hospital.

Mack hurried to meet them. "What have you got?"

"A vehicle rollover ending in a fire. Patient is nonresponsive."

He swallowed. Anything involving fire reminded him that Theresa was still in the hospital mourning the loss of her baby. She'd regained consciousness in time to say goodbye to her infant, but once the physical pain of her treatments wore off and she had time to think, it would probably all hit her.

He checked his patient's pupillary reflexes and swiftly moved to check other vital signs as the gurney was wheeled toward a room.

What if Theresa had been Lainey and he hadn't been able to make things right?

The problem was, Mack didn't know how to do that.

Glenda's comment had made him delve into

the reasons behind his reaction. It was because of his own childhood of being dragged around the country over and over. He saw Lainey's decision to move to Boston, and now possibly somewhere else, as a repeat of what he'd endured.

But he was a grown man now, not a child. There was no school to be pulled out of. No friends that he would completely lose touch with—not in this day and age of social media and instant access to people via text or a phone call. He wasn't in danger of losing anything. Except the woman he loved.

And yet never once had he congratulated her on being given what amounted to a huge promotion and an acknowledgment that her skills were exceptional.

He'd never once offered to go with her or even visit her. And in all that time, he'd never contacted her once. He'd deserved to be kicked to the curb. Forever.

And yet she'd offered him what looked like a second chance, and he turned around and did to her what he'd felt she'd done to him those years ago. He'd discarded her without even asking for an explanation.

"I heard about the accident." Rhett swept into the room as he and a nurse were getting an IV started. "Anything I can help with?"

A huge wave of grief overtook Mack that had nothing to do with his brother or the patient and had everything to do with the possibility that he might lose Lainey a second time. Just as they were starting to fall in love again. At least he knew he was in love with her.

"A rollover ending in a fire. They got him out before he got burned." He ran down the man's vitals, ending in, "Rhett, can you take the lead on this one? I have to step out for a bit."

His brother took one look at his face and said, "Go. I've got this."

"Thanks. I owe you."

"Remember that when it comes time to decide who gets the position." He made a face. "I'm kidding, Mack. Go deal with whatever it is."

"Keep me updated."

He nodded. "Will do."

With that, Mack swept out of the room, discarding his gloves in the nearest receptacle and heading to his office. But once he got off the elevator on the second floor and let the doors close behind him, he stayed where he was.

Hiding in his office and brooding would not solve anything.

But he knew what might.

Turning around, he pressed the button that

would call the elevator back. And then he headed down to the first floor.

Lainey was in the break room eating a cinnamon roll when she sensed someone standing there watching her. She glanced up. It was the very person she'd just vowed to hunt down and demand an explanation from. He looked pretty imposing, with one hand braced against the doorjamb, clicking and unclicking something on the wall with his thumb.

She wasn't sure why, but she'd decided today was the day she was going to find him. Originally she thought she'd wait two weeks to confront him, but she couldn't wait that long. Not this time. She wanted things settled before she decided things for sure.

Lainey had taken another look at those job offers, and although none had stood out to her, she needed to at least weigh whether she could work in the same town as Mack. And she thought she'd come to a decision.

"Mack. What are you doing here?"

"I'm actually looking for you. Can I join you?"

She shrugged. "Suit yourself. There's not much left other than cake type stuff."

Well, that wasn't a very nice way to greet

him. Not when her heart was about to pound out of her chest at the sight of him.

“I’m not here for food. I’m here for you.”

If her heart was struggling to fly free before, it was positively banging at the bars of her chest now, trying to break out of its cage. “Me?”

He sat across from her. “I realized something today. I never told you I was proud of you when you were approached for the job in Boston. I am. Very proud of you. Even though I didn’t act like it.”

“Thank you.” His words surprised her. She’d actually never thought about that before. She allowed herself a trace of hope, that this might be the chance she’d been hoping for on their last night together.

“You deserve every good thing that life hands to you, whether it’s here or at one of those other places.”

Her heart stopped pounding at the bars and slowed down. Maybe this wasn’t going to be an “I Love You” speech. Maybe he was going to say goodbye—or he needed to have a sense of closure this time that he hadn’t gotten before.

“Are you hoping I’ll take one of those jobs?”

He looked at her for a long moment, and she wanted to cry. But she held herself together. Somehow. Now was not the time for emotion. She could fall apart later. After he was gone.

"Would you ask me to come with you?"

Had she just heard him right? Hope dawned once more, then another thought torpedoed it yet again. "Is this because of the baby?"

"No." There was no hesitation to his response. It was as if he knew the question was coming. "I'm doing what I should have done two years ago. Celebrating your accomplishments and joining you in them."

"But your job…"

"I can work anywhere. I could even open my own practice if I wanted to."

She was shocked. What had changed between Boston and now? "But why?"

"I don't want to lose you. Not again," he said simply. "I love you."

Those three words came out of the blue and hit her right between the eyes. There was no beating around the bush this time or making her guess his meaning—he'd stated it in no uncertain terms."

"God, Mack." She was so afraid. So afraid this was going to all blow up in her face again. "Are you being serious? Because if not, you need to tell me right now."

He scooted his chair close to hers and then used his finger to tilt her chin up. "I've never been more serious about anything in my life. I've made a lot of mistakes. But believe it or not, I think I've finally learned from them. Tell me it's not too late."

She leaned forward and pressed her face into his shoulder. "It's never too late. As long as we're breathing. I love you too." Lainey reached for him and kissed him, a long kiss that was punctuated by the sound of a door opening and then slowly closing again with a quiet click of the latch. Whoever it was had stuck their head in and then left again.

If she'd been hoping to keep the baby's paternity secret, she had a feeling that had just been blown out of the water. But she didn't care.

She finally came up for air and opened her eyes, so glad to find this wasn't a dream. It was reality. *Her* reality.

"So where are we going?" he asked.

"Well, we could always do my place again if—"

He laughed. "I like that idea, but I meant more along the lines of where in the United States."

"As far as I know, nowhere. But you'd really go if I decided that one of those jobs looked interesting?"

"I really would. Austin hasn't been home for quite a while. At least until you came back. I know now you're not like my dad. You won't make decisions without thinking about both of us. And I'll no longer expect everything to be a repeat of my childhood."

She knew what he meant. Because she'd done the same. "I promise the same thing. I promise to try not to see things through the filter of how I grew up. And I'll try not to act like requests are orders that must be resisted."

"You? No." He said it with such sardonic drama that it made her laugh.

"I said 'try,' I didn't say I'd always succeed."

"Got it." He kissed her again. "Do you know if you want to stay at the clinic or do you want to come back to the hospital?"

"But Glenda said..."

"I know what she said, and I know I have a decision to make about whether Jack or Rhett gets the position, but for now, I want to kiss the woman I love and ask her to marry me again."

"Yes."

His brows went up. "I haven't asked you yet."

"I'm being proactive rather than reactive, remember? This is part of my new mission statement. Yes. I'll marry you again. The sooner, the better."

"I agree. And since we already have the baby furniture set up at the apartment, we can live there if you want to."

She remembered saying she didn't want to live anyplace more permanent. Lainey had made her share of mistakes too, including making Mack feel uncertain of how important he was in her life.

"After what happened to Theresa and her baby, I don't think I can stay there and look at that damaged block and remember what happened. Can your place hold all of us?"

"For now. And if it gets too small, we can relocate. Anywhere you want."

"How about anywhere *we* want. Let's vow to make this a true partnership this time. You, me and Annabelle."

"No, not Annabelle. She gets no vote in this matter." He laughed before cupping her cheeks. "In all seriousness though, thank you. For loving me enough to give me a chance to make things right."

"Oh, I know you're going to make things *right*…once we get back to my place tonight." She frowned. "Speaking of making things right. Have you thought about trying to figure things out with your brother and your dad? And maybe even reaching out to your half sister?"

"Actually, my dad reached out to me yesterday and wants to talk. I said yes. As for the rest, I promise to work on my family relationships. After all, if I was given a second chance with you, anything's possible."

"Oh my goodness, I love you, Mack Morrison. More than you'll ever know."

"Pretty sure I love you just as much." He waggled his brows. "So when does your shift end?"

She glanced at her watch. "In about fifteen minutes. Why, what do you have in mind?"

"So many things. And the first of them involves getting you home and out of your clothes."

Her teeth came down on her lower lip before releasing it. "I bet I could get Sofie to let me off a few minutes early."

"I can wait fifteen minutes."

"But I'm not sure I can. Besides, we've been quiet for the last hour, and I'm pretty sure that was my replacement who came in here a few minutes ago, probably looking to see what goodies had been put out."

"Well, let's go ask her."

"Let's do it." She snickered. "And then we can *do* it."

"For as long as we want?"

"For as long as we want." She reached up to kiss him. "I love you."

Together they walked out of the break room hand in hand to find a line of clinic staff outside the door. They all clapped in unison, including Sofie.

"Sorry," Mack said. "We didn't mean to take up the whole break room."

"Don't say sorry. But maybe next time turn off the intercom before having one of your special chats." She reached in and flipped a toggle switch that was sitting right where Mack's hand had been when he was standing in the doorway. Lainey remembered him clicking something repeatedly with his thumb.

"Oh Lord." She laughed. "So I guess you all know who the father of my baby is?"

"We do. So do all of our patients. And it sounds like you're headed home to plan your next few arrivals."

Lainey smiled and lifted her chin, not at all embarrassed. Actually, she was proud that someone like Mack wanted to be with her, even after everything that had happened. And she promised herself that she'd make sure he knew it each and every day of their lives.

* * * * *

Look out for the next story in the Paging Dr. Morrison duet:

Doctor's Nine-Month Rival
by Kristine Lynn

And if you enjoyed this story, check out these other great reads from Tina Beckett:

Nurse's Second Chance at Forever
Expecting Her Best Friend's Baby
Second Chance in Santiago

All available now!

Now, read on for an tantalizing excerpt from
Nurse's Second Chance at Forever
by Tina Beckett

Nurse Louisa has a "no bad boys" rule. Her daredevil ex's death in a racing accident made sure of that. Now, facing the future as a single mum, Louisa's trying to put her shattered heart back together. Until the arrival of ER doc and adrenaline junkie Dane has her skidding off course. Even one scorching look from him sets her body alight! But when Louisa learns Dane is fighting his own demons, it's not just temptation that draws her to him, but their once-in-a-lifetime bond…

CHAPTER ONE

DANE CRIGHTON HAD been doing chest compressions for five minutes straight. He knew that because the newest member of his team kept on giving him a countdown after each minute had passed. Her voice was right in his ear, the headsets necessary to combat the noise of the chopper, but he found it distracting, even though he knew it was standard protocol for their air rescue squad. Most people knew that he wasn't fond of the constant reminders, however. Dane was able to keep a mental countdown that helped him keep track of how long he'd been going.

"Let's switch."

This time he frowned. This was the second time she'd offered to take over, her Southern drawl identifying her as being from a different part of the country. Dane was well aware that CPR fatigue was a real thing, but he worked hard even on his days off to keep himself up to par in the stamina department for just this reason. But it would interfere with his concentration if he had to keep telling her he was fine, especially since this time she hadn't phrased it as a question.

He glanced at her, aware that it was more of a glare before saying, "Okay, switch."

She ignored the pointed look. As if perfectly synchronized, they switched positions, with Dane now on the Ambu bag and the nurse doing compressions. And her rhythm was spot-on. He'd found himself critiquing each and every thing she did. He wasn't sure if it was because she was new or because something about her vaguely irritated him. Maybe it was her self-assurance. Maybe because he'd noticed her in a way that was other-than-professional ever since they'd first been introduced yesterday.

Today, her hair was pulled up in a clip, one dark strand falling free and bouncing to each timed thrust of her hands. Something about that caught his attention and fascinated him, although his mental computer of what they needed to do to save this man's life still worked flawlessly in the background.

Their patient was thirty-four year old Matt Harrison, who'd suddenly collapsed while hiking in a more remote area of Flagstaff with three buddies. One of them had thankfully started CPR immediately while another called 911. Because of the terrain and distance to the nearest hospital, it was decided to airlift him out rather than try to evacuate him by rescue squad.

Dane's gaze flicked to his watch, and because he knew she was expecting that countdown, he said, "One minute."

They'd tried defibrillation and two doses of epinephrine, and they'd gotten him back once, only to have him revert to V-fib.

They were still a few minutes from landing at Flagstaff Memorial, where they could do more diagnostics to try to figure out how to fix the problem. Matt was young, and Flagstaff's cutting-edge cardiac care unit was his best shot at a decent recovery.

"Two minutes."

He had to admit, the new nurse was making CPR look easy. Her cheeks were flushed, but she kept counting, the numbers sounding as strong as when she'd started.

He squeezed the Ambu bag twice for every thirty compressions and glanced again at his watch. Fifteen seconds left. The second hand slowly moved forward until it was time. "Three minutes. Let's reassess, then switch."

He knew she would immediately agree, as opposed to him. She seemed to be a by-the-books player. Not that this was a game. It was deadly serious.

Just as she stopped compressions, Dane was surprised to hear a blip on the heart monitor. He held his hand up in a signal to wait as his gaze jerked upward to the readout. Holding his breath, he watched as the familiar cadence of a true sinus rhythm scrolled across the screen. It was followed closely by a couple of chaotic beats, but then seemed to settle back in. When he glanced at his partner for this trip, he saw she was also staring at the monitor. Neither of them moved for close to a minute.

The rhythm stayed in place, and Dane blew out an audible breath, a sense of exhausted relief washing over him. Getting out his stethoscope, he placed it against the patient's chest, even though he knew the odds of the machine malfunctioning were almost nil. The second dose of epinephrine they'd given at the five-minute mark had evidently taken a little longer to act than he'd expected. But at least it had kicked in. Now they just needed to land. And that steady beat needed to stay in place.

As if reading his thoughts, the chopper pilot's voice came through his earpiece, letting them know that they were getting ready to land at the hospital. He saw the nurse's lips move as if praying. Or maybe she was just breathing out a thank-you to the universe. Whichever it was, he sent up one to add to hers just as he felt the helicopter's landing gear touch down on the helipad.

Even before the rotors had finished powering down, a team of three people burst from the doors of the hospital, wheeling a gurney. He recognized one of them as the head of cardiology who had received national recognition for tweaking the way valve replacement surgery was done. He'd transferred from one of the country's top teaching hospitals, saying he'd needed a slower pace for the sake of his family. Dane had overheard the term *silver fox* used by one of the nurses in the ER when talking about the surgeon. But if Jake Norden was aware of those whispers, he gave no sign.

All he knew was that their patient was damned lucky to have landed on Flagstaff's doorstep.

"Hi, Dane. What have you got?"

He gave Jake a rundown on what had transpired as they transferred the patient to the gurney and power-walked back to the hospital. He was vaguely aware that the nurse who'd been on the flight was following behind at some distance as if she felt her part in the patient's care was done. As if relegating herself to a lower spot on the team. But that didn't settle right with him.

"Can you keep me updated on his condition?"

"Sure thing. Thanks." With that, Matt's new team bustled through the door, bypassing the ER and heading straight to the elevator, where they would undoubtedly go to the cardiac wing on the second floor.

Dane waited at the door, holding it open for the pilot and the nurse, who were walking together, talking about the case. He'd tried to remember her name the whole flight and had come up empty. Something that wasn't like him either.

He could blame it on swearing off relationships after a recent breakup had ended up… well, volatile on his ex's part. But that didn't mean it was okay to brush off niceties, like learning someone's name.

The pilot smiled. "Well, Lou, welcome again to Flagstaff Memorial. It was great working with you."

Ahhh, that was it. Her name was Louise. Or was it Louisa?

"You too. Thanks!"

Chuck, the pilot, nodded at him as he walked by. When the nurse followed, Dane said, "Er… Lou, could I speak with you for a moment?"

Her eyes widened, and a trace of uneasiness entered her gaze. “Sure. Is something wrong?”

Now that he had her attention, though, he wasn’t exactly sure what it was he wanted to say. But he gave it his best shot. “No. Everything’s fine. I just wanted to thank you for what you did up there.”

Her brows went up, and her lips curved slightly. “You mean…for doing my job?”

But that sexy accent held no hint of reproach, so at least she didn’t think he was being an ass. At least, he hoped not. He felt one side of his mouth twitch up in response. “I just didn’t want to breeze past you without at least saying something. Do you want to grab a coffee?”

And why he’d asked that, he had no idea. He decided to tack on some kind of explanation so she didn’t think he was hitting on her. He definitely wasn’t. “I don’t know about you, but my adrenaline is always pumping after every rescue.”

This time she laughed. And that low-throaty sound…something bottomed out in his abdomen.

“So you’re going to add caffeine to the mix?” One of her brows arched.

He smiled back. “Doesn’t everyone?”

“Not me, but to answer your question, yes. I

could go for something, sans caffeine. Is there a cafeteria in the hospital?"

"Yep, just off to our right." They started walking. "Do you prefer Lou? Louise?"

"Lou or Louisa is fine. Most people just call me Lou, though."

"Okay, Lou it is. And you can call me Dane."

"Dane. Sounds good." She glanced at him as they walked. "How long do you normally perform CPR?"

"As long as it takes. Why?"

"No. I mean, do you have a preferred length before you hand off to someone else? I noticed you didn't want to switch that first time. And since we'll probably be working together on runs, if we're both on duty when the call comes in, it would be nice to know."

He'd been kind of gruff the first time she'd offered to step in, and he knew it. "Sorry about that. I can normally do two or three cycles without fatigue setting in."

"I see. Is that what you prefer to do?"

"It is."

They made it to the cafeteria and got in line, which wasn't as long as it could have been. He ordered an espresso, and Lou ordered a frozen decaf coffee drink. When the attendant asked if she wanted any flavoring in it, she asked if they had mocha.

"We sure do." The young guy behind the counter gave her a brilliant smile, and Dane almost rolled his eyes. He was probably all of eighteen, and Lou had to be at least… He wasn't going to touch that. Not that she looked like she was out of her teens herself, but to become a critical care nurse took a few years. So he was betting she was in her early thirties.

They got their drinks, and Dane sat down at one of the tables that had a view of the San Francisco Peaks in the distance. She glanced out and took a drink of her coffee. "This is so different from Alabama."

Her voice was soft, almost as if she was mulling something over.

"Ahh, that explains your accent. What part of Alabama?" It was normal small talk that usually meant nothing, but he found he was interested. Flagstaff probably did seem different from the Southeast.

"About fifty miles east of Birmingham." This time she looked at him but didn't offer anything more or the name of the actual town.

He didn't want to pry, so he offered up another question instead. "That's quite a journey. How did you decide on Flagstaff Memorial?"

"Actually, I needed a change, and I saw the ad posted in an online nursing journal."

"So you applied."

She smiled again, and this time the curving of her lips hit him somewhere in the midsection, setting off a warning bell in his head. He needed to be careful. Jana had left a bad taste in his mouth—her expectations of what a relationship should be had been far beyond what he was willing or able to give—and the last thing he wanted was to give off vibes that signaled interest.

"I did. And the rest is history, as they say."

"How do you like it so far?"

"The hospital is great, but Flagstaff itself isn't how I pictured it. I thought there'd be long stretches of desert and hundred-degree temperatures."

"We don't get as hot as other parts of Arizona, but we are in a drought and have been for a while. July usually brings monsoon season, which helps, but it evaporates so quickly that in recent years, it hasn't raised the water levels by a whole lot."

She looked out the window again. "Well, it's beautiful. And…it's not Alabama."

Said as if that were a good thing. But this time, he decided to just let that go without commenting on it.

"Well, I'm glad you like it here."

"I do, so far. We'll see when the school year rolls around if that continues."

When he tilted his head in question, she went on. “My daughter will be starting kindergarten this year. Another reason I thought this was a good time to move.”

His eyes went to her left hand. No ring. And the skin on her ring finger wasn’t any lighter than the rest of her hand.

Divorced? Or just a single mom?

None of his business. And he’d do well to remember that.

“I see. I hope she likes it.” He downed the rest of his espresso in one swallow and set the cup on the table.

“So do I.” She gave a shrug with one of her shoulders. “My in-laws weren’t super happy about my leaving, but… I just couldn’t stay under the circumstances.”

So maybe it was a divorce situation. Another reason to be thankful that he and Jana had broken it off before having kids, which she had been pressing for recently. But he hadn’t been ready, and he wasn’t sure why. Maybe because his own upbringing had been fraught with conflict, his mom doing her best to police his activities and control what sports he could participate in. Just like she’d done with his dad. And Jana…well, she’d given off some vibes that made him wonder what their future would be like. Whatever the reason, he was happy with his life the way it was. And it was certainly different from the corporate life his dad had led. But Dane wasn't interested in sitting behind a desk. He was a self-proclaimed adrenaline junky, and emergency medicine suited Dane's personality to a T. He shook himself back to the present, remembering what he was going to say.

"I'm glad you landed at Flagstaff. You're certainly good at what you do."

"Thanks. It's a little different from my last position, since my former hospital didn't have an air rescue unit. But I talked to a friend who was involved in CareFlight, which is one of the major air ambulance services in my area of Alabama, and she loves it, so I decided to take the plunge."

That surprised him. He assumed that she *had* done it at her last job, since she'd seemed at ease with the confined space and didn't seem nervous about being in the chopper. "You must not mind air travel."

"Air travel, no. But skydiving or anything involving being in the air while outside a plane, yes."

"So no hang gliding or parasailing for you."

"Nope to both of those. You?"

Dane happened to love hang gliding, but he could understand why a lot of people were afraid of the sport, especially here in Flagstaff. The only good launch site was on Mount Elden, and wind conditions and landing could be tricky to navigate. Jana hadn't been thrilled with him going up.

"I've done both and enjoy them."

Something in her face changed. Grew harder, if he was reading her right. But he wasn't sure why that would be. Maybe her ex had been a hang glider?

He didn't even know if she had an ex. She hadn't referred to her in-laws as "former," so maybe she wasn't divorced. Again, not his business.

He decided to try to end their conversation. He needed to get back to the ER anyway. "I'm sure plenty of people will offer, but if you ever have any questions about Flagstaff, feel free to ask. I was born and raised here, so I'm pretty familiar with the ins and outs of the city."

"Thanks, I will. At the moment, though, I need to go and finish out my shift. I'm sure I'll see you around."

"I'm sure you will."

With that, she got up and threw her trash in the receptacle, while he bided his time by pretending to answer messages on his phone so they didn't have to leave together. He wasn't sure why, though. The ICU wasn't on the ground floor, so they wouldn't actually be headed in the same direction. Maybe it was the way she made him feel off balance, as if he couldn't figure out what she was thinking. Or maybe it was just that damned accent. And the nagging wonder if it deepened while in the midst of…

Oh hell, he'd never find that out, so why did it matter?

It didn't. But now that the thought had been birthed, it was going to be hard as hell to get rid of it. Still he waited until she was out the door before he tossed his own trash and headed back to the emergency department—a place where things were rarely ever dull. Just like hang gliding. Or dirt bike courses.

And that's the way he liked them.

Don't miss
Nurse's Second Chance at Forever
by Tina Beckett

Available wherever
Harlequin Books and eBooks are sold.